D1825237

Mastering the Marketplace: Taking Your Practice to the Top

Ross D. Clark, DVM

With original and reprinted material provided by

Marty Becker, DVM
J. Tol Broome, Jr.
Tom Carpenter, DVM
Tom Catanzaro, DVM, MHA
Dennis Cloud, DVM
Brad Coody, MBA
Jan Coody, MBA
Thomas G. Diffell, DVM
David B. Goodnight, DVM, MBA
John Lofflin

Dave Madden, JD
Will Novak, DVM, MBA
Ron Patrick, MBA, CPA
Kirk Putman, CPA
Paul M. Schmitz, DVM
Carin A. Smith, DVM
W. Bradford Swift, DVM
Dave Watson, CPA
Ron Whitford, DVM
Fritz Wood, CPA

Veterinary Medicine Publishing Group, Lenexa, Kansas

© 1996 Veterinary Medicine Publishing Group

Published by Veterinary Healthcare Communications, formerly
Veterinary Medicine Publishing Group
8033 Flint, Lenexa, Kansas 66214; Web: www.vetmedpub.com

First printing: 1996
Second printing: 2001
Printed in the United States of America

Library of Congress Catalog Card Number 96-060136
ISBN 0-935078-57-6

Acknowledgments

I would like to thank my brother Delbert, a large-animal veterinarian, and sister-in-law Marilyn for taking me in every summer from the ages of 10 to 18. It was there that I developed my love for veterinary medicine. I would like to thank all my other brothers and sisters—Betty, Lawrence, Loral and Edward—and their families, who helped raise me after our mother passed away when I was 10.

I want to thank Drs. Roy Millerette and Bruce Wren at Kansas State University for making my summer job as a student assistant in the necropsy room enjoyable. Drs. Allan Bradbury and Joe Wagner at Gage Avenue Animal Hospital in Topeka also made veterinary medicine fun; my thanks to them as well.

I first heard about Dale Carnegie and the mental side of practice and life through Dr. Jake Mosier. I thank him for always being an extremely positive role model.

As a new graduate, I moved to Chicago and worked with two more veterinarians who loved veterinary medicine—Drs. Ken Bone and Bill Barnes.

I next worked for Dr. Ray Russell in Mesa, Arizona. There I learned more about pride and love for our profession and gained further insights into the principles of veterinary practice management.

To recent or soon-to-be graduates, I recommend that you carefully pick your first jobs based on your perception of the quality of medicine practiced there and the positive tone of the owners, associate veterinarians and other staff members. Your level of financial success, as well as the quality of medicine you practice, is very likely to be a mirror image of that first practice.

When I came to Tulsa—where a high percentage of practices were American Animal Hospital Association (AAHA) members—veterinarians like Drs. Ed Hoffman, Bob Featherston and Glen Harbert preached and practiced high-quality, ethical veterinary medicine. Without their idealistic examples of conservative veterinary medicine, my natural enthusiasm for marketing might have drifted toward a more competitive format too early in the evolution of practice management.

I want to thank my partners—Jim Osborn, Dennis Henson, Pat Grogan, Jan Coody, Ron Hooley and Mike Jones—for their belief in me as the manager of the group of practices known as Woodland PetCare Centers, and for allowing me to do what I love—be a full-time administrator and philosopher.

Many thanks to Dr. Paul Schmitz who converted all my long-hand notes and facilitated correspondence between contributing colleagues and our office. Thanks also to Betsy Leedy for helping bring the book to completion when Paul left for Chicago in the summer.

I also want to thank my lifelong friend Bob Myers, who always sees the opportunities and the positive outcome of the marketing and management ideas that I propose.

A big thank you to my wonderful wife Linda and the rest of my family—Brad, Sheri, Kent, Kimberly and grandson Kash—for their patience and support.

Last of all, but not least, I want to thank Dr. Ray Glick, Rebecca Turner, Renée Anderson, Peggy Shandy, Dr. P. Lynne Stockton and all the staff at Veterinary Medicine Publishing Group.

Sincerely,

Ross D. Clark, DVM

Preface:
Some Opening Thoughts

by Ross D. Clark, DVM

I appreciate your buying this book. If you want to peruse the contents and quickly page through whichever chapters immediately catch your eye, I encourage you to do so! If you want to start with the introduction and read through page by page and chapter by chapter, that will work as well.

This book is replete with practice management tips. You might want to read with felt-tipped highlighter in hand. Its accompanying *Practice Workbook* provides an exercise for giving your own practice a quick checkup, innumerable forms you can reproduce for use in your practice, sample contracts, marketing texts and guides to goal setting. You may want to do as I do. I use the insides of the front and back covers and the table of contents pages (with the page numbers) for making notes for later consultation. As a result, I can reread the book in just a few minutes by reviewing these highlights!

I encourage you to make these books living documents ... filled with my ideas, my contributing authors' ideas and your own ideas and/or goals. This book could be worth many thousands of times the purchase price if you turn these ideas into actions.

Only 10 percent of Americans write down their goals annually. A mere three percent write down their goals annually, review them regularly and develop a five-year plan. These few people who write down, review and update their goals on a regular basis accomplish more than the other 97 percent combined.

Contents

Chapter 3: Financial and Strategic Planning

Chapter 4: Marketing, Advertising and Public Relations

Chapter 5: Medical Records

Chapter 6: How to Work with Banks and Credit Bureaus

Chapter 7: Partnership and Associate Agreements

Chapter 8: Leasing, Buying and Selling Practices

Chapter 9: Managing Miscellanies

Chapter 1:
Practice Performance

Call to action

by Ross D. Clark, DVM

"An unexamined life is not worth living."

Plato

   Changes in veterinary medicine, and all professions, are occurring on organized and unorganized levels. According to Bob Anton, CEO of Veterinary Centers of America, our profession is presented with a changing paradigm as many different groups attempt to carve their own niches in our profession.

   Changes have been documented in human medicine, and we can learn by looking at the human health-care scene. The central hospital is being partially replaced by cancer care centers, surgery centers, diagnostic imaging centers, radial keratotomy centers, rehabilitation centers, sports medicine centers, industrial medicine centers and plastic surgery centers, to name just a few. These centers now compete with central hospitals in every city. They are owned and operated by everything from multinational corporations to groups of local doctors joined together to form local corporations. As a result of this competition and specialization, many central hospitals have been forced to close.

The human medical industry is now shaped by health maintenance organizations (HMOs) and similar large corporate entities. They tell people which clinics, hospitals and doctors they can use. Ninety-five percent of today's doctors get their patients from contractual referrals. Veterinary hospitals have begun to consolidate and "pet super stores" are reshaping our industry.

General small-animal practice owners are being pinched on three levels: at the top by the ever-increasing numbers of board-certified veterinarians, in the middle by "niche" practices and at the bottom by discount vaccination clinics and low-cost spay/neuter clinics.

Daniel Yankelovich, a premier pollster, said in the October 5, 1992, issue of *Fortune* magazine that the formation of public opinion on important issues resembles a biological process, evolving slowly through seven clearly defined stages: After a (1) dawning awareness that a problem exists, (2) comes a sense of urgency, (3) then the discovery of choices, (4) wishful thinking, (5) the weighing of choices and finally, (6) the taking of an intellectual stand and (7) the making of a responsible judgment.

The small-animal practitioner, in competition with Big Business for the position as gatekeeper of veterinary medicine, has been through at least the first four of these seven steps. Wishful thinking, however, will not pay any percentage of the rising costs of doing business. Big Business will surely leave these practitioners behind if they don't decide what tools they need for carving their niches in this extremely complex and competitive race.

Such tools include learning how to attract and motivate quality-conscious clients, offering clients options instead of standard procedures and possessing the best technology available. At the same time, we must not move away from client contact. Mrs. Clark is far more concerned about how "Misty" reacts to you and your hands than in how adept you are at surgery.

Leaders produce change; they don't run from it. They see change not as a threat but as a challenge. If you wish to retain the position of gatekeeper, remember that leadership is an attitude and a state of mind.

We at Woodland PetCare Centers of Oklahoma faced the same challenges as the rest of the industry. We decided to become more pro-active in the face of a pet superstore with its accompanying seven-days-a-week, full-service veterinary clinic and seven-days-a-week grooming services. Our practice had been doing well: gross was up, numbers of transactions were up and dollars per average transaction were up. In spite of this nice growth, our net income as a percentage of gross had declined for the sixth quarter in a row. We were now down about 1.75 percent as a percentage of net to gross. I called my entire staff to action with the following document. The results were astonishing. Our net income as a percentage of gross increased eight percentage points from our low, resulting in a 40-percent increase in net income.

Clear and present danger: Superstore opens within one mile...

CONFIDENTIAL: TO ALL EMPLOYEES

We have learned that a national chain will be opening a second facility, a large pet superstore/veterinary clinic, one mile away from our central hospital. This now presents us with a superstore within one mile of four of our five Tulsa locations. The superstore will be open seven days a week and will offer evening hours, low-cost vaccinations and low-cost spays and neuters in their full-service veterinary medical clinic. They will spend thousands of dollars in advertising on their Grand Opening weekend alone. They have every right to be here and to compete for pet-care dollars. This is the beauty of America and the free enterprise system.

Each year that goes by finds me thinking that Woodland PetCare Centers will reach critical mass as the number of new referral clients consistently exceeds clients that move away. This year, at last, total transactions, average transactions and gross income are all up. However, net income as a percentage of gross has been declining for the second year in a row. This may result in part from our lower-priced vaccination clinics and from holding the line on other prices while our costs continue to soar; however, this lost income alone does not completely explain our lower net income. We must constantly be more efficient and cost-effective to compete in the new world of veterinary medicine.

How do we turn this clear and present danger around?

In recent months, I have reviewed hundreds of publications—including *Harvard Business Review*, *Fortune* and *Forbes*—to learn what businesses are similarly experiencing declining net incomes and increasing competition problems and to learn what their solutions are. It gives me little comfort to know that veterinary medicine is not alone. Here's what I found:

Challenges:

First: Change occurs at a frantic pace out there in the business world, leaving seemingly invulnerable companies, hundreds of times bigger than ours, dazed and perplexed.

Second: Computerization has so far failed to deliver decreased costs and increased productivity, although it has enabled us to access volumes of valuable data that we would not want to live without.

Third: Clients/customers are smarter and more demanding than ever.

Fourth: Companies that retain employees also retain customers. For example, banks and auto dealerships, two businesses abysmally poor at building customer loyalty, are also abysmally poor at retaining employees. In contrast, at Woodland PetCare Centers, blessed with experienced, long-term staff, we are currently attracting more clients than we are losing.

Fifth: It is no longer effective to offer to "make it good" or "fix it for nothing." The new client wants it done right the first time. Busy schedules do not allow time for return visits to "fix it." Return visits to fix things not done right the first time cost us money and reflect badly on our professionalism. We need to do things right the first time. We must become a "zero defects" company to ensure near "zero defectors" from our client base.

Solutions:

Renew: To ensure our survival, we must create a company prepared for constant renewal and constant improvement. We must work very hard to retain the clients we currently have, while constantly reinventing our company through new services and new technology. The Japanese have a word for this process of constant renewal and reinventing. They call it *kizan*.

Focus: We must align our aggregate thought processes around common objectives through monthly staff meetings and weekly committee meetings. An organization such as ours must renew and reevaluate our mission/vision statement. This will give us a competitive advantage over less-focused competitors.

Visualize: According to Warren Bennis—a psychologist, sociologist, economist and University of Southern California professor who has spent years studying corporate chiefs—"A leader is the person with the indispensable first quality of having a guiding vision ... a clear idea of what he or she wants to do and a plan to get it done."

Listen: From our focus group studies, recently completed by New City Marketing, I propose we develop a client service department at the receptionist desk. We will staff this area, as much as economically possible, for constant and instant feedback on our service satisfaction level.

Benchmark: We must establish a disciplined way of measuring our performance. We must "benchmark" against AAHA's "practice edge" management reports and against other successful practices in our practice management study group. We must continue to monitor, through information obtained by New City Marketing and our client service staff, our clients' perceptions of the quality, speed of delivery and value of our services.

Tools:

Teamwork and empowerment: Management will solicit more active collaboration of all staff members in continuously finding better ways to do things. We will work harder on developing quality communication with staff members so that they may be informed and empowered enough to deliver quality timely services to our clients.

Gemini Consulting's Four R's: Gemini is a global management consulting firm that specializes in business transformation. It has over 1,700 consultants and 16 offices on four continents. Its managerial director, James Kelly, believes companies fail because they try to effect too many changes through unfocused efforts. Kelly says, "If real change is to occur, company owners must first establish a framework for transformation by determining the purpose of the program, its expected benefits, the resources committed to it, and the allotted time frame."

Gemini Consulting has identified "Four R's of Business Transformation:"

1. *Reframing*—adopting a strategic vision, making it an integral part of the cultural mindset and mobilizing the organization for change.

2. *Restructuring*—continuously adjusting the business portfolio to keep resources strategically placed and re-engineering the process to ensure maximum efficiency and continuous improvement.

3. *Revitalizing*—inventing and growing new businesses.

4. *Renewing*—participating in strategic alliances (e.g., PennHIP®, ICG®), partnerships, joint ventures and other collaborations; and growing the organization's people through re-skilling, re-deploying and leveraging technology to accelerate their rate of learning.

Work with suppliers: In the world of change, few industries are changing faster or more profoundly than health care. Traditionally, drug and supply sales representatives called directly on doctors to discuss the benefits of new products. Now they meet with committees of physicians and business administrators of large buying groups. Not only do the products have to meet medical standards, but they must also meet profit standards, either individually or through increased sales of related products.

We must communicate our problems to our suppliers and work with them as a team in order to lower our cost and provide quality, fresh products to our clients.

Be client-oriented: Are some of our clients more equal than others? We must become a client-based company with consistent improvements in our service. Tom Peters in his recent book, *The Tom Peters Seminar*, tells us that the question every company must now ponder is: "Who will testify to your need to exist during the last 12 months?"

We need to find the real magic of client loyalty. If we can put that magic to work for us, a beneficial flywheel effect will kick in, powered by repeat sales and referrals. Revenues and market share will grow. Steady clients/customers are easier to serve than are new clients/customers. They understand our mode of operation; but when they ask for help, we had better come running. A study done by the Bain Company estimates that a decrease in the customer defection rate by only five percent can boost profits by 25 to 95 percent. The Bain Company says that we cannot learn much about our clients with a simple customer satisfaction survey. In the restaurant business, *60 percent of the customers who end up defecting typically describe themselves as satisfied or very satisfied.*

Satisfaction surveys are good for openers and for the vanities of company owners, but quality and value ratings are better indicators of customer retention. Customers who have had problems solved are more loyal than those who didn't have a problem at all. We must continue to do whatever it takes to rapidly resolve client problems.

We must focus our company's resources and attention on that 20 percent of our clients that bring us 80 percent of our gross income. First, we must identify those loyal clients and make them members of some special club—not to receive more discounts, but to receive more service and direct contact—like newsletters, birthday cards, special seminars and other benefits Team Woodland will develop at our next series of staff meetings.

We have sold these people on our professionalism. We need to involve them in our clinics so they will carry our professional banners into the marketplace among the purveyors of pet food and low-cost vaccinations.

Jack Smith's turnaround tips: Jack Smith became CEO of General Motors in 1992. By July of 1994, he had not only stopped the bleeding of that "Rust Belt" giant, he had engineered the biggest turnaround in American corporate history. General Motors' incredible turnaround violates the conventional wisdom of a generation of business people and academics. Here are Smith's turnaround tips:

- Establish a vision for the whole company.

- Set clear expectations for performance at each level of the organization.

- Construct realistic strategies that don't require rocket science.

- Develop the capability to execute by reorganizing people and reallocating assets.

- Focus everything—all assets, all decisions—on your customers ... the ultimate arbiters of success or failure.

Peter Senge's five disciplines: Peter Senge writes in his best-selling book, *The Fifth Discipline Fieldbook, Strategies and Tools for Building a Learning Organization* (New York: Doubleday, 1990) that a learning organization always evolves.

Senge thinks competitive advantage is derived from continued learning, both individual and collective. This makes sense, but it won't happen unless members of the organization go through personal transformations.

No more thinking that we have all the answers. We must learn and master new scientific management tools like ladders of inference and systems thinking, personal mastery, mental models, shared vision and the fifth discipline—team learning. Senge's five disciplines boil down to the assertions that people should:

1. put aside their old ways of thinking (mental models);

2. learn to be open with others (personal mastery);

3. understand how the company really works (systems thinking);

4. form a plan everyone can agree on (shared vision); and then

5. work together to achieve that vision.

A nine-step game plan

As I noted above, our bottom-line turnaround was dramatic. Here is a nine-step game plan to take your practice to the top.

1. Develop a SWOT team of five to 10 staff members to review the practice, identifying its

   Strengths,
   Weaknesses,
   Opportunities, and
   Threats.

   a) Review Chapter 1 together. Develop a prioritized list of company goals.

   b) Communicate company goals to staff members by making an intense commitment to regular staff meetings.

   c) Develop a mission/vision statement for your hospital or clinic.

2. Develop a discipline to hire carefully and train extensively. Keep employees long-term. Chapter 2.

3. Develop financial and strategic plans that guide in the creation of realistic budgets and attainable missions. Use proactive pricing. Benchmark against the best. Chapter 3.

4. Develop comprehensive public relations, marketing and advertising programs. Chapter 4.

5. Re-evaluate your medical record keeping. Make sure your methods support your procedures and protocols. Get ready for electronic medical records. Chapter 5.

6. Assure your continuing access to credit and capital with solid financial reports, winning business plans and accurate credit reports. Chapter 6.

7. Pick associates and partners carefully. Negotiate with them fairly and honestly. Tie down your understandings with contracts and partnership agreements. Chapter 7.

8. Maintain and enhance the physical plant and equipment that support your practice. Pick good locations. Negotiate favorable leases. Chapter 8.

9. Tend to the details. Manage the miscellaneous. Chapter 9.

How healthy is your practice operationally?

by Ross D. Clark, DVM

The premium veterinary hospitals are those leaders that constantly learn from their experiences. They readily discard old ways of doing business and create new and effective strategies. I call that the Learning Imperative. To learn more about the health of your practice, use this quick practice health checkup.

I'm sure you routinely recommend annual exams for your patients. Well, turnabout is fair play. It's time to follow your own advice and conduct an annual checkup of your practice. If you use your computer to monitor progress, you have access to financial data that will tell you where you've been ... and where you need to be.

To determine if your practice is as healthy as it should be, I suggest you scrutinize your operating efficiency, practice goals, training and marketing programs, reminder system and building maintenance. Here's how:

Ideally, you should record sales and production figures for each profit center in your practice and for each associate as well. If you use incentive programs, you can also track the sales figures of your paraprofessional staff and then compare employees' performance records. The following surveys will help you evaluate your practice. As you read about each measurement, think about how well your practice meets the outlined goals. Then turn to the *Practice Workbook* and take the Quick Checkup in Section 1: Practice Review.

How efficient is your operation?

If your practice's gross revenue and net profit figures look great to you, keep in mind that those numbers may have been accomplished at the expense of your practice's long-term success, even if they fall within national averages. For example, a high net may result from high fees but an inefficient staff; or it may result from low fees but an overworked and underpaid staff. In either case, your practice could be headed for trouble in certain areas.

Do you need to realign your staff? To decide, consider the following two calculations:

- The total number of hours worked, divided by the total number of client transactions.

- The employee costs, divided by the total number of client transactions.

These formulas include all practice employees, including associate veterinarians and owner veterinarians; but you may want to calculate the figures separately. For example, let's say Hospital A has 10 full-time nonveterinarian employees who work 1,730 hours a month, the total monthly nonveterinarian employee expense is $10,380 and the hospital records show 1,000 client transactions per month.

According to the first formula, this practice spends 1.73 nonveterinarian staff hours per transaction per month (1,730 ÷ 1,000). According to the second formula, the nonveterinarian employee cost is $10.38 per client transaction ($10,380 ÷ 1,000).

Formula 1:

Total staff hours ÷ Total client transactions = Total hours per transaction

_____ hours ÷ _____ transactions = _____ hours/transaction

Formula 2:

Total staff costs ÷ Total client transactions = Total cost per transaction

_____ costs ÷ _____ transactions = _____ cost/transaction

Now let's suppose that the three veterinarians at Hospital A work 45 hours a week each, or 193.5 hours a month (based on 4.3 weeks a month), and that each veterinarian averages 333.3 client transactions a month. Two of the veterinarians earn $46,000 a year; the third earns $28,000. Total veterinarian salary expense: $120,000 a year, or $10,000 a month.

Going back to our formulas, we find that the hospital spends 0.58 veterinarian hours per transaction ([193.5 x 3] ÷ [333.3 x 3]). Based on the second formula, the veterinarian cost per transaction is $10 ($10,000 ÷ [333.3 x 3]). Hospital A then shows 2.31 total employee hours per transaction (1.73 + 0.58) and a total personnel cost of $20.38 per transaction ($10.38 + $10).

Now for the analysis: Initial surveys indicate that 1.5 personnel hours per client transaction is about average. As you can see, Hospital A is operating inefficiently. What about the cost per transaction? Determining an average is difficult because of the wide range of fees charged nationwide. One way to appropriately use this number, however, is to remember that total employee costs (veterinarians and nonveterinarians) should not exceed 43 percent of your gross practice revenue or 43 percent of your average charge per transaction (ACT). Therefore, if Hospital A has a $60 ACT, it can support a personnel cost of up to $26 per transaction. (For more on calculating productivity, see Chapter 7, "Associate compensation.")

Of the two calculations, I find personnel hours per transaction to be the best measurement of practice efficiency. Why? Because by looking at the total number of personnel hours per transaction, you take salary and fee considerations out of the equation. Thus, you can fairly compare a practice in "Big City," USA, to a practice in "Small Town," USA.

How realistic were last year's goals?

Most practice owners want their bottom line to be in the upper five percent of the national net income surveys. Sometimes the raw materials just aren't there to achieve such results. For example, if your area is in a recession or if the local population is declining, increasing your profit is more of a challenge ... but it's not impossible. The way to start is by setting realistic goals for gross sales and net profit and then monitoring them regularly. It's also important to establish for your practice a clearly defined mission and a budget, each of which will help keep your goals on track.

How effective is your training program?

Today, a well-trained staff isn't a luxury; it's a requirement. New clients see and assess your staff long before they rate your expertise; and if they haven't been treated in a professional, friendly and positive fashion, they certainly won't be in the mood to accept your recommendations. Good client relations are based on trust and the feeling that you care for your clients' pets as much as they do. To make certain your staff understands the level of commitment you expect, create a written job description for each position in your hospital, including technicians (kennel, lab and surgical), receptionists, cashiers, veterinarians and interns.

I also recommend that you assign a mentor to each new employee, perhaps a senior employee or an associate. You may want the mentor to be in charge of assessing the new employee's progress, but the most important aspect of the relationship is that the mentor be someone from whom the new employee can learn without being intimidated or feeling intruded upon.

Another valuable tool is a training video that new employees can take home or watch in a quiet room in your hospital. After several screenings, staff members should understand the basic functions of their jobs, including your expectations, the reasons why things are done the way they are at your hospital and the employee's role in the overall scheme of client satisfaction. Our practice produced its own training video, but commercially produced videos are available as well.

Bear in mind that if your employees perform tasks their own way rather than the way you want, utter confusion will result. Clients will quickly get the message that no one knows what's going on. Your goal should be consistent, reliable, high-quality service in a friendly yet professional atmosphere. As international consultant Bob Beale says, "The tiebreaker is customer service, so get clear in your mind what customer service looks like through the customers' eyes."

At Woodland PetCare Centers, we've witnessed the benefits of dedicated and hard-working employees. That's why we devote at least one percent of our annual gross revenue to quality employee training.

How efficient is your reminder system?

The most important client-targeted piece of mail you send is the vaccination reminder. In these days of soaring postal costs, however, your reminder system may need a face-lift. The days of nickel postcards are gone, and even 20-cent postcards can add up to a sizable sum in a year's time.

To ensure that your reminder system is as efficient and cost-effective as possible, your receptionists and cashiers should be trained to keep the client files in the computer up-to-date. Every time mail is returned because of a wrong address, the correct information should be entered both in the computer and on the patient chart.

Also, be sure to note in the computer and on the chart when a patient dies. Few situations are as embarrassing as hearing from a sobbing client that she has just received a vaccination reminder for the cat you euthanized last week.

You also should take a look at the time frame you're covering and the response you're getting to your second and third reminders. To track them, keep a record for three or four months. You may discover, for example, that clients are coming to you for everything but routine vaccinations, particularly those clients on fixed incomes. If reduced-cost vaccination clinics are readily available in your area, your clients may be patronizing them. In response, you may want to offer once-a-week or even daily "value vaccination" clinics. Keep in mind that the objective is to serve these clients and save them money without lowering your fees for the bulk of your client base.

You also may decide to send only two reminders. If so, the first should be targeted for due dates up to 30 days from mailing; the second should target those patients with vaccinations up to 30 days overdue. Or, after you've made sure these clients are still active, you may want to substitute a letter for the second post-card. A letter allows you to convey your concern that the pet isn't immunized, specify what can happen to an unprotected animal, offer a "value vaccination" day or send a personal note.

Whatever reminder program you choose, be sure to send out reminders every month, without exception. There's no reason every client shouldn't get a timely vaccination reminder. Remember, it's the most important piece of mail you send a client, because it's the one that will reap the most return.

How effective is your target-marketing program?

Your high-tech equipment and well-trained staff won't do you much good if no one knows where your practice is. In this age of media hype, you have to do what you can to compete for your share of potential clients' attention. When you develop your budget at the beginning of each year, be sure to devote some money to target-marketing programs.

Which practice promotions should you highlight during the year? There are numerous options. For example, February is a good dental-health month; spring is a good time to introduce heartworm and flea-prevention programs; and summer opens up the potential for increased boarding opportunities and dog dips.

Target-marketing examples:

- Design messages that welcome new clients and thank clients for their referrals.

- Consider making contributions in memory of deceased pets. This helps bond clients to your practice,

- Send messages recommending dentistry or suggesting spays/neuters.

- Send breeders a special newsletter, provide puppy or kitten packs and discount certificates for their customers, or offer special rates on pet foods or services. After all, breeders' referrals are very important to your practice.

- Use your computer to sort and select for all manner of groups, classes and breeds; and send a letter to one group a month, explaining the origin, expected behavior and potential medical problems of that particular breed or type of pet.

- Generate other computer lists, such as a birthday list for the pets that belong to your most loyal clients. They'll love the idea that you know Spot's birthday and care enough to send him a birthday greeting.

- Generate a computer list of your top 100 clients and send them greetings for Christmas, Hanukkah or other holidays, while at the same time thanking them for the opportunity to be their veterinarian.

Whatever you do, be sure to target some type of mailing—other than reminders—to at least one section of your client base every month. Keep in mind that no one knows your clients better than you do. That's why you should select the kind of programs and promotions that your clients will appreciate, and choose as many as will fit your budget. Remember, your practice's target-marketing program is only as limited as your imagination and your budget!

> *Whatever you do, be sure to target some type of mailing—other than reminders—to at least one section of your client base every month.*

How well is your building maintained?

Does the building reflect good taste and suggest that your hospital is prosperous and open for business? Maintaining your facility means more than taking out the trash and sterilizing your instruments before everyone goes home at night. Is your building a pleasant place to enter even when the smiling faces aren't there? When you open the door from outside, what do you smell?

It's easy for us to acclimate to the smells of dip, kennels, accidents on the carpet and wet dogs. Clients aren't accustomed to these smells, however, and don't want to smell them. That's why you should make sure your air-freshener system is operating effectively ... even if your system consists only of a kennel technician armed with air spray and fresh mop water!

Now take a look outside. Is your parking area clean or is it littered with soft-drink cans and cigarette butts? It really doesn't matter who made the mess; if it's in front of your door, make sure someone is responsible for picking it up ... every day!

We pay a premium wage for the time one of our employees spends picking up trash. Even an older building can be spruced up to look new and pleasing to the eye. For example, at Woodland PetCare Centers, our natural dark rock was the latest trend when we built the facility 20 years ago; but we've since painted this rock a contemporary off-white to gray, and now it looks great!

Six time-honored *abilities* of practice management

This is an easy-to-remember list of time-honored marketing and management ideas that may exist within your comfort zone but not within your practice.

The debate over the professionalism and effectiveness of managing and promoting your practice is likely to continue into the 21st century. Whether you stand firmly in the "professionalism camp" or in the camp that says veterinary medicine is a business and should be run like one; or even if you try to somehow straddle the fence, there is still common ground in the field of marketing and managing. All veterinarians should carefully monitor these two camps if they wish to be successful. Use this checklist of *Ability Factors* to gauge how effectively you are directing these noncontroversial aspects of marketing and managing your practice.

In 1963, Dr. Leroy Atkinson, a highly successful veterinarian in St. Louis, Missouri, told me about three *Ability Factors* of practice success. The first of these is Avail*ability*. At the time I visited Dr. Atkinson, he lived next door to his clinic and had one veterinarian actually living in the clinic. The other two factors he introduced to me were Ami*ability* and plain old *Ability*.

All three of Dr. Atkinson's *Ability Factors* have proved helpful to me. In their broadest interpretation, they cover the essentials of practice management. Over the last 32 years, I have added three more *Ability Factors* to the list: Cred*ibility*, Adapt*ability* and Vis*ibility*.

Ability factor #1: Availability

How easy is it for your clients to do business with you?

1. How often do callers get a busy signal when trying to reach you? If it is often, then it isn't very easy for them to schedule an appointment. For around $65 you can find out for sure by ordering a "busy study" from the business

office of your phone company. This study will tell you how many times a day your phones give would-be callers a busy signal. If you average more than two "busys" per hour, you should add a line as soon as possible. Contemporary telephone systems can also give you an accounting of incoming and outgoing phone calls by each individual telephone and by total calls.

2. How many hours per week is your practice available to your clients? In this changing society, we are faced with increasing numbers of clients who simply cannot get to the clinic during traditional office hours. When both spouses are working through lunchtime, evenings and weekends may be their only scheduling opportunities. A recent AVMA study indicated that 31 percent of all pet-owning households consider convenient office hours to be an important factor in choosing a veterinarian.

3. Is there plenty of clean, well-lighted parking near your front door? If there is, then you have an ideal situation and your clients don't need to worry about whether they will find a place to park or whether they will make it to your door safely. Negative thoughts and concerns about accessibility can build up subconscious resistance to returning to your hospital. If you don't have an ideal parking situation, you're probably painfully aware of how difficult it might be to change that. But don't give up easily. Study the problem. Discuss it with your associates and employees as well as with your clients. Brainstorming might just provide the creative solution you've been looking for. When one West Los Angeles veterinary hospital ran out of parking, they hired two valet parking attendants.

4. Does your clinic take its own emergency calls? Utilizing an emergency clinic is a mixed bag. On the one hand, you and your staff have the opportunity to be better rested and therefore better prepared to take on the day. Morale

is likely to be higher, and you might even be able to maintain a higher quality of medicine. On the other hand, there are costs for such benefits. Not only is there a loss of emergency income, but there is the loss of long-term income from potential new clients. One way to get the best of both worlds might be to take your own emergency calls until midnight. In my experience, people rarely notice (and almost never cause) life-threatening conditions in their pets when they are in a state of slumber. Therefore, the odds are in your favor that you would capture the lion's share of the night's emergency cases before midnight and still get a good night's sleep.

5. What ancillary services do you offer your clients? When attending to their pets' needs, clients tend to seek the path of least resistance. They may "think" they're happy dealing with separate businesses for pet food, boarding, grooming and veterinary care; but what happens when they run across a facility that takes care of everything with one stop? In our present society, time is becoming more and more important.

6. Which credit cards do you accept? Do you accept Visa, MasterCard, Discover and American Express? This is your best method of low-risk credit management. By accepting all cards, you are providing options your clients will appreciate. For example, when a client has reached his or her limit on one card because of a recent major purchase, you can offer the flexibility of permitting the client to use another card. You are also making it easier for your clients to pay you, even when they "forget" their checkbooks or don't bring enough cash.

Ability factor #2: Amiability

How enjoyable is it to do business with you?

Every time you walk through a door, you are subconsciously wondering what kind of experience you are about to have. Every positive experience in a location reinforces your desire to return to that place. People generally gravitate toward cheerful and courteous people because they have an expectation of a positive experience. These are basic psychological premises ... but what are you doing to create them?

1. How pleasant is your staff? This may sound like a silly question; but if you listen to your staff answer the phone or greet clients, you may be surprised at what you hear. But don't stop there ... How pleasant are you? How excited or genuinely pleased are you when addressing clients? Sincere smiles and warm greetings might be the most valuable acquisitions your hospital could make this year.

2. What kinds of signs greet your clients and prospective clients when they walk in the door? *"No Credit," "We Reserve the Right to Refuse Service to Anyone," "You Will Be Charged Extra ...," "No Hospitalized or Boarded Animals Will Be Released When the Doctor Is Not In," "No Refunds"* are examples of negative signs that can give clients the subconscious feeling that they are a nuisance to you. There are positive professional ways to deliver most important messages. For instance, you could change *"No Smoking"* to *"Thank You For Not Smoking!"* Try to limit your signs to a few well-worded messages. This will not only increase the effectiveness of the messages, but it will reduce the feeling that your office is cold and impersonal.

3. Is your clinic free of offensive odors? Steps must be taken to seek out and destroy all odors that your clients might find offensive. If your clinic smells like a fresh and clean home, you'll make a lot of points with your clients. The

sense of smell has a much more powerful and long-lasting impact than sight.

4. How would your clients describe your reception area? If the process of waiting to see the doctor is the most nerve-racking part of an office visit, then you have a problem you can do something about. What is it? Is the reception area chaotic? Are pets crowded too closely to each other? Are cats upset about dogs? Are kids running around uncontrolled? Is there not enough seating? Whatever the problem is, find it and reduce or eliminate it!

5. How long do your clients have to wait before seeing you? What can be done when you have a full appointment book, and then constant walk-ins gum up the works? Short waiting times are obviously desirable. Apart from providing the usual complement of magazines and plenty of seating, there are ways to cut down both actual and perceived waiting times.

    a) Some practices have had success with continuous-loop videotapes that entertain clients as well as educate them on light veterinary topics.

    b) A glass display case can also entertain and educate clients if it is set up as a mini-museum, containing interesting objects relating to veterinary medicine (such as foreign bodies that have been removed from patients).

    c) Escorting clients into exam rooms the moment the rooms become available gives clients the feeling that they are progressing, and sometimes the move resets their internal clocks. Research shows that today's client has an internal clock of eight minutes before he or she becomes uptight; but each time you pay attention to the client, you gain another eight minutes of his or her patience. After you have the client settled in the exam room, if you measure and record this wait, you and your staff will become much more aware of the value of your clients' time and will have a measure for minimizing future waiting times.

6. Do your clients sometimes experience difficulty carrying food, supplies and pets back to their cars? The full-service gas station may have died out at one time, but it is making a comeback with firms like Autograph® and Pep Boys® that feature uniformed attendants who do everything from auto detailing to checking fluid levels to filling your tank with gas. Society is now placing a higher value on service. Most of your clients are willing to pay for service extras; and if you don't offer them, they may seek someone who does.

7. Is free coffee service available to your clients? Not only does this please your coffee-drinking clients, but it helps provide a pleasant aroma to your reception area.

Ability factor #3: Professional ability

How is your professional image?

Ability is a subjective matter. You have very few opportunities to demonstrate your actual ability to your clients, so they judge you every day upon whatever they observe. If they are going to judge your professional ability by the color of your shoes, I suggest you choose your shoes wisely.

1. Do you and your staff look professional? Clients' perceptions of professional credibility take a big positive jump when veterinarians wear clean, white labcoats. The VMI (Veterinary Management Institute at Krannert School of Business, Purdue University) says that a white lab coat rates 17 percent higher than any other uniform choice. When you provide your staff with matching smocks or uniforms with name tags, you are distinguishing them as a

team of professionals. When each staff member wears a name tag printed in large, easy-to-read letters, your clients can get to know each member of your team ... an important factor in building a lasting bond. By including the team member's title on the tag, you are building staff pride and job satisfaction as well as client awareness of the many functions performed by your staff. It is also a good idea to identify new trainees with name tags so that beginners' errors and slow service do not reflect badly on the entire staff.

2. Do your dispensed items look professional? Are your prescription labels typed? Are prescriptions dispensed in a safety vial? Professionally dispensed medications convey your professional image to clients' family members who weren't able to visit your hospital.

3. Are clients aware of your fees? Do you freely offer estimate slips for more involved cases? Some of your clients may be apprehensive about a treatment plan because they overestimate its cost. If you ease their minds, they just might open up to your plan. On the other hand, if they are underestimating, it is even more important to let them know costs up front. The fewer surprises you give your clients, the fewer they will give you when it comes time to pay!

4. Do all new clients go home with a clinic goodwill kit? These kits usually consist of pet food and vitamin samples, care guides and other assorted goodies inside a colorful plastic sack. Most clinics I know give such kits to their clients with new puppies or kittens, but what about such a package for those with new adult pets? Free goodies provide an excellent way to build goodwill and get a new client/patient relationship off to a great start!

5. Are the public areas clean and well decorated? Dirty floors and peeling paint are indications to the client of

your professionalism and caring … or lack thereof. It is amazing how a can of paint or a roll of wallpaper can improve your image … as well as your staff's attitudes!

6. What are you doing to help your clients learn more about their pets? Many clients crave an understanding of what caused their pet's illness, what you are going to do about it and how they can prevent it in the future. Satisfying their craving for knowledge will create a lasting bond. Handouts created in-house are more personal and tend to have a bigger impact than those provided by a vendor. Train your staff so that they feel comfortable instructing clients on the proper use of all of your over-the-counter (OTC) products and on proper pet care.

7. What are you doing to help your clients learn more about your services? If you are like most of us, it's probably not enough. You might be quite surprised to learn how few clients know you offer boarding or dentistry. Some might even have taken their pet to a spay/neuter clinic not because it was cheaper, but because the name made them realize that the service was offered.

It may sound farfetched to change the practice name to include all the services you offer, but I do suggest that you examine your "practice awareness" campaign and look for ways to improve it. Try offering clinic tours, providing a hospital brochure with pictures, hanging pictures of the rest of the clinic in the reception area. A client questionnaire can educate your clients on your services while providing you with valuable information about how well you're doing. Just asking your clients to indicate which services they have received and which services they are aware that you offer, is a means of telling them what you offer.

Ability factor #4: Credibility

How is your reputation within the community?

No matter where you live, your market area is likely to have an unwritten code of expectations for veterinarians. If you want to maximize the opportunities available to you, it might be wise to try to identify those expectations and heed them.

1. Is your lifestyle consistent with acceptable behavior in your area? If your community is very liberal, then a traditionally conservative lifestyle might not "fit in." For example, if there are strong animal rights sentiments in your area, then hunting and fishing might not be the best way to spend your spare time. If you choose to do so anyway, at least keep your treasured mounted trophies out of your place of business. As they say, "When in Rome..."

2. How is your work-ethic image? A regular golf game and liberal vacations may be well deserved; but in some rural areas, they may be hard to justify if you want to charge higher than average fees.

3. What about your image for honesty and integrity? In this profession, nice guys finish first. Doing business like J.R. Ewing of the TV series *Dallas* may produce short-term gains, but it might also be hurting your practice more than you realize.

Ability factor #5: Adaptability

How sensitive are you to changes in the profession and your market area?

Obviously, the way veterinary medicine is practiced today is quite different from the way it was practiced even 10 years ago. These changes take place through advances in medicine and changes in client needs. Most practitioners tend to fall into one of three categories when it comes to new ideas. They lead; they follow, or they get in the way. I suggest you not do the latter!

Ability factor #6: Visibility

How aware is the community of your clinic's existence?

There are many ways to keep your name and your clinic's name in the public's eye:

1. Write articles. Many cities have neighborhood papers eager for regular columnists. Timely pet-care articles are always popular.

2. Provide trophies or veterinary services to local dog and cat club events, shows and matches.

3. Offer a meeting room (if available) at no charge to dog and cat clubs.

4. Send marketing letters (e.g., newsletters, breed letters, birthday cards).

5. Offer a Pet Transport Van displaying the name and number of your hospital, to help maintain top-of-the-mind awareness.

How healthy is your practice financially?

by Ross D. Clark, DVM

"It pays to own up to mistakes as soon as possible."
Bruce Nyland, Reflections for Managers

Practice managers and owners customarily have monitored key expense areas known to management aficionados as the "big three"—supplies (including drugs), rent and personnel. But as our profession continues to experience consolidation, as more and more partnerships and corporations comprise multiple hospitals employing more and more non-owner veterinarians, it is increasingly evident to me that we should now be tracking the "big five," to which we can easily apply the "big five formula"—20-20-20-20-20. That is ...

- twenty percent or less for cost of sales for drugs, supplies, pet food, lab work and dead animal pick-up;

- twenty percent or less for veterinary staff salaries, *including* a salary for owners or partners;

- twenty percent or less for non-veterinary staff salaries and benefits;

- twenty percent or less for rent, marketing, advertising and public relations, including 10 percent or less for rent and 10 percent or less for the rest; and

- twenty percent or more for profit, bonuses or retained earnings—depending on the type of business (partnership, corporation, etc.).

Of course these are only guidelines. A new practice may spend more than 10 percent for rent, but should compensate with lower veterinary personnel costs. A more mature practice may be able to keep rent costs as low as four to six percent.

Practice managers and owners customarily have monitored key expense areas known to management aficionados as the "big three" — supplies (including drugs), rent and personnel.

A mature practice may have a total non-veterinary personnel cost of 24 percent, but should be able to lower veterinary costs to 16 percent or lower for a maximum staffing cost of 40 percent.

Cost of sales may vary because of the mix of your practice. If you do more boarding or grooming, then the cost of sales should decline while personnel costs increase because those activities increase the cost of labor rather than the cost of goods sold. If you do major amounts of grooming, then grooming should be treated as an individual profit center.

It may also be helpful to track your practice's key financial ratios and compare them with the national averages and medians for veterinary clinics provided in the the following pages as well as in the accompanying *Practice Workbook*'s Section 1: Practice Review section.

Key financial ratios

Liquidity or solvency

Liquidity measures the short-run ability of a practice to pay its current liabilities.

Net working capital: excess of current assets over current liabilities.
Formula: current assets minus current liabilities = net working capital
National average = 42,000*

Current ratio: measures short-run debt-paying ability.
Formula: Current assets divided by current liabilities
Of course there are a few practices with minimal to zero current liabilities.
National range and median = 1.0 to 5.5, median is 2.5*

"Acid test" or quick ratio: measures short-term liquidity.
Formula: (current assets minus inventory plus net receivables) divided by current liabilities
The ultimate liquidity test, this ratio recognizes that inventory is not totally liquid, although this formula retains receivables as a fairly liquid asset.
National range and median = 0.5 to 3.0, median is 1.5*

Profitability ratios

Profitability ratios measure the financial soundness of a business.

Return on sales: indicates profits earned per dollar of sales.
Formula: net profit after taxes divided by sales
This ratio measures the efficiency of the operation.
National range and median = 1.8 to 18.2, median is 10.6*

---

*Ranges and medians shown here were calculated from a combination of information from Dunn and Bradstreet, AAHA reports, Robert Morris and Associates, Practice Management Edge and my personal experience as a consultant.

Return on assets: matches net profits with the assets available to earn a return.
Formula: net profit after taxes divided by total assets
This ratio indicates a clinic's profitability.
National range and median = −1 to 16.3, median is 6.9%*

Return on net worth: matches profitability and equity.
Formula: net profit after taxes divided by net worth
This ratio provides a means of analyzing the clinic management's ability to realize an adequate return on the capital invested by the owners of the clinic.
National range and median = 5.3 to 46, median is 22*

Efficiency ratios

Inventory turnover: acts as a speedometer on the clinic's merchandise.
Formula: sales divided by inventory
This ratio indicates the rate at which merchandise is being moved and the effect of the flow of funds into a business.
National range and median = 19.4 to 63.4, median is 39.8*

Collection period: acts as a speedometer on the clinic's receivables.
Formula: (accounts receivable divided by sales) multiplied by 360
Reflects the average number of days to collect receivables.
National range and median = 3.9 to 20.8, median is 12.2*

Accounts payable to sales: measures the extent to which suppliers' money is being used to generate sales.
Formula: accounts payable divided by sales
When this ratio is multiplied by 365 days, it reflects the average number of days it takes the company to repay its suppliers.
National range and median = 1.1 to 3.9, median is 2.4**

** Veterinarians do not typically report monthly accounts payable to banks and other survey companies.

Assets to sales: relates assets to sales.

Formula: total assets divided by sales

This rate ties in sales and the total investment in assets that is used to generate those sales.

National range and median = 13.3 to 47, median is 23*

Sales to net working capital: acts as a sort of efficiency meter for the clinic.

Formula: sales divided by (current assets minus current liabilities)

This ratio measures the efficiency of management in its use of short-term assets and liabilities to generate revenues.

National range and median = 8.6 to 26, median is 17*

Dunn and Bradstreet information services offers a new report called "Business Scope" that will compare your clinic or hospital in all the above categories, plus many more. You could also compare your PAYDEX score. The PAYDEX system analyzes the payments in their file for a given business and converts that record into a numerical score. PAYDEX scores are updated daily and are based on as many as 875 trade experiences for a single business. The PAYDEX is tracked over a full two-year period along with industry norm scores for comparison and trend evaluation.

You may also benchmark your numbers against other hospitals by subscribing to the AAHA "Practice Management Edge Reports." The advantages AAHA reports have is that they compare by region and by size of practice.

Preventing practice failure

by Marty Becker, DVM

With the competitive pressures facing veterinarians today, it's no wonder so many practices struggle just to stay ahead. It seems no matter how many positive changes we make, the competition keeps picking up speed in a never-ending race toward success. In today's veterinary marketplace, a major mistake could leave you behind—or put you out of the race altogether.

To keep your practice healthy, it's important to take a *preventive* approach to problems. Examining the most common reasons small businesses fail is a positive first step. Why? Because doing so is likely to reveal your practice's vulnerabilities and to provide valuable insight into what will better enable you to succeed.

> *To keep your practice healthy, it's important to take a preventive approach to problems. Examining the most common reasons small businesses fail is a positive first step.*

Why do small businesses fail? Michael Gerber, author of *The E-Myth: Why Most Small Businesses Don't Work and What to Do About It* (Harper Business, 1990), recently released his list of the 10 top reasons small businesses fail. Does your practice show any of these deadly symptoms?

1. *Lack of management systems.* It's no secret we didn't learn about management in school—or that there's still relatively little business instruction in the schools today. But veterinary practice is a boat with two oars—one representing clinical skills, the other, business skills. Those of us who don't learn to keep both oars in the water, rowing simultaneously, will find ourselves going in circles. Resisting the need to learn about business is a sure path to failure.

2. *Lack of vision and purpose.* Many practices cling to the status quo, imitating others and providing only basic services. While looking to the past won't save you from failing, a clear purpose for the future just might. Every practice needs a powerful, positive, proactive vision that is talked about, taught and personified by everyone involved.

3. *Lack of financial planning and review.* Are you still lamenting the slow winter of last year or planning for the winter ahead? Remember, just because your practice isn't sick doesn't mean it's healthy.

4. *Overdependence on specific individuals.* Many practitioners fail to delegate enough responsibility to others, holding their practices hostage to low productivity. Another related mistake: Failing to cross-train staff members adequately.

5. *Poor market segmentation and/or strategy.* The best strategy in today's crowded veterinary marketplace is to foster the perception that your practice is unique. How? By constantly giving your clients what they want and what their pets need *before* they look for it elsewhere.

6. *Failure to establish and/or communicate your practice's goals.* Setting goals and measuring progress are the most important steps in realizing your dreams for your practice. As Sandy Ogg, Via Consulting Group Inc. in San Diego, says, "Make sure your mission and goals are in the halls—not just on the walls."

7. *Competition and a lack of market knowledge.* Sadly, the days of mom-and-pop businesses are numbered. To be successful today, business owners must have state-of-the-art "systems-training;" and they must understand the market to compete effectively.

8. *Inadequate capitalization.* Management consultant Dr. Gerald Snyder, Boca Raton, Florida, notes that "most veterinary hospitals are only one month's cash flow away from major, often fatal, consequences." Are your practice finances under control? *Now* is the time to find out.

9. *Absence of a standardized quality program.* Consider the saying: "Some succeed because they are destined to. Most succeed because they are determined to." With a standardized quality program in your practice, you can work to be your best and, eventually, you'll be among the best.

10. *Concentration on the technical, rather than the strategic, work at hand.* I recently saw a wall plaque that says: "We cannot direct the wind, but we can adjust the sails." Practice owners are harbor pilots who help steer their practices through uncharted or turbulent waters.

It's okay to fail *forward*

I'm not suggesting you should never fail; in fact, if you aren't failing, you're not moving forward. As educator John Condry said, "Setbacks often lead to innovation and renewed achievement." The key is to prevent your practice from experiencing a "fatal" failure.

At a recent veterinary meeting, several management consultants agreed that veterinarians will fail in direct proportion to their:

- tendency to resist change;
- failure to adapt to change; and
- willingness to blame such outside forces as competition.

Successful practitioners *embrace* change by anticipating what tomorrow's clients want and what their pets need—and by taking personal responsibility for the outcome. Financial guru Charles Given sums it up best: "There are unlimited excuses for failure, but no one ever makes excuses for success."

Success is a journey

In the next few years, I believe we'll see the veterinary battle-field littered with dying practices. Most of us felt secure in the old environment; we believed the profession would remain stable and prosperous. But let's face it: People will never stop wanting better services, better products and better lives—and they'll tolerate no less from veterinary medicine.

Despite the changes, however, our profession *can* build upon a solid foundation of traditional strengths and a great reservoir of public trust and admiration. Empowered by passion or a vision, we must use faster, more flexible, higher-tech tools to build and maintain successful practices.

To set your practice on the right path, look past the obvious and concentrate on the *potential*. Just as you would consult reference materials or experts to help diagnose and treat your patients, you must look beyond your ZIP code to cure management ills, prevent problems and optimize your practice's health. It is much easier—and more enjoyable—to keep a healthy practice successful than it is to cure an ailing one.

This article first appeared as "Why veterinary practices fail—and how to protect your own" in the July 1994 issue of *Veterinary Economics*. It is reprinted here by permission of the publisher.

Top consultants spot problems and opportunities

by Fritz Wood, CPA; Dave Watson, CPA; and Kirk Putman, CPA

In 1993, Hill's Pet Nutrition, Inc. commissioned consultants from Arthur Andersen, the world's largest management consulting firm, to assess the problems and identify opportunities for small-animal veterinary medicine practices. The results of this study have been so appreciated by practicing veterinarians and Hill's that additional consultation to the veterinary profession is ongoing. The following recommendations are taken from an article that appeared in the November 1993 issue of Veterinary Economics*:*

We recently completed a profitability study of small-animal veterinary hospitals. What did we learn? Plenty!

For one, we were surprised by the profits and incomes veterinarians generate. Given the academic demands, we expected to see much higher income levels. For the same reason, we also expected to see a fairly low level of business savvy among veterinarians, and our findings confirmed that expectation. The good news? We see great opportunities for improvement and success in veterinary practice.

What's missing?

Before we look at the opportunities, let's take a look at some of the problems. We found, for example, that many veterinarians fail to:

- understand that veterinary medicine is, first and foremost, a service business;

- understand or embrace the concept of "creating value in the eyes of the client;"

- appreciate the importance of the "client experience;"

- market their services effectively or make their services more appealing;

- shift work from peak periods to off-peak periods;

- delegate work appropriately to qualified staff members;

- see that veterinary medicine is a fixed-cost business, and understand the implications of operating in that environment;

- focus on cash flow instead of "mark up;"

- understand or embrace the concept of inventory turnover; or

- recognize the contribution to profits generated by over-the-counter sales.

Bottom-line opportunities

Please don't misunderstand us. As business consultants (and consumers of veterinary services), we appreciate all that is "right" with your profession. Our goal here is simply to communicate what we see as incredible opportunities to improve your financial performance—especially bottom-line results and take-home pay.

We believe, for example, that most veterinarians truly endeavor to offer the highest quality care to their patients and clients. We also believe that financial success allows you to practice that desired level of care. If you don't enjoy some degree of financial success, you can't afford the facilities, staff and equipment required to deliver the best care. Financial success is nothing to be ashamed of—it's the vehicle required to realize your dreams and to fulfill your obligations to your profession.

What would we do?

We've been asked what we would do if we owned or managed a veterinary hospital. Although we don't claim to know all of the answers (or even all of the questions), we would make sure that our veterinary hospital had:

- A pleasant and inviting appearance and aroma.

- A happy, friendly, caring, gentle, sincere and genuine staff—both face-to-face and on the telephone. The first and last person the client sees leaves the biggest impression, so we wouldn't tolerate dullards.

- Convenient office hours that accommodate two-wage-earning and single-parent families.

- On-schedule appointments and minimal waiting times.

- Services and products that emphasize convenience and "one-stop shopping."

- Client-feedback mechanisms to make sure we provide what clients want, not just what we think they want.

To keep the practice healthy and successful, we would:

- Find ways to continuously learn more about our clients—their wants, needs and expectations.

- Retain key employees to minimize turnover.

- Actively solicit referrals and reward clients who refer others.

- Aggressively make call-backs to comfort clients and to encourage compliance with recommended procedures and the home use of prescribed products.

- Practice good medicine by recommending the necessary procedures. We wouldn't predetermine a client's ability or willingness to spend money on a pet.

- Charge premium fees for our outstanding services.

- Carefully capture and collect charges for *all* services rendered.

- Make sure our well-trained (and cross-trained) staff did everything except diagnose, prescribe and perform surgical procedures. The doctors would spend their time on value-added work; that is, work that clients are willing to pay for and that advances our business financially. Before our doctors would do anything, they'd ask: "Can someone else do it?" They would thus have time to examine more patients every day.

- Actively identify and communicate opportunities to perform ancillary services (e.g., geriatrics, dentistry), then perform them, especially in off-peak periods throughout the year.

- Make sure our clients would say "yes" if they were asked: "Did you have a good time at the veterinarian?" Whoever said visiting the veterinarian *shouldn't* be fun? In all seriousness, this question is being asked about physicians—who are frightened by the answer and its implications. Medicine doesn't have to be cold, sterile or impersonal. Pet owners have a choice. And as most are incapable of discerning medical competence, they can only assume their pets are treated the way they are.

- Create an annual business plan and regularly check our progress. Why? Because if we don't know where we're going, we won't know when we get there. We'd factor in inflation and expected productivity gains, and wouldn't be satisfied with the same or lesser results than the year before.

- Encourage everyone on staff to practice self-improvement, whether it be through reading, taking classes at the local community college or completing vendor education programs. We'd read business and management books and magazines, and implement or enhance good ideas from others (both within and outside the veterinary profession).

- Insist on continuous improvement through aggressive goal setting and focus on those things under our control. For example, we know we can't control the incidence of disease, but we can control prevention. We would carefully track our progress on the percentage of puppies and kittens receiving all of their immunizations; puppies receiving heartworm prevention; animals receiving annual fecal analyses; adult dogs receiving annual heartworm checks; clients receiving and complying with nutritional counseling; animals receiving dental prophylaxis; older pets receiving geriatric exams; and clients complying with other recommended services.

- Recognize our staff members' contributions and implement their suggestions.

A real-world example

Enough rhetoric; it's time for a concrete example. Let's assume we operate a practice in a community that requires annual rabies immunizations. Let's also assume we have intense competition from vaccination clinics offering $10 immunizations. Should we throw up our hands, decide not to compete and abandon the profession? Not if you work in our hospital.

The first step is to create a strategy for success. But how can we differentiate this service? After all, aren't immunizations a commodity? No way. Commodity is a state of mind. That means we face the competition head-on, even though we're smaller and don't have deep pockets. We know which business has the stronger relationship with our clients, and it's *not* Vaccinations-R-Us.

So, first we identify our slowest month of the year. Then we send a letter to all of our clients inviting them to visit us that month to take advantage of a special offer: We will perform a complete physical examination and give a *free* rabies vaccination. The total cost for this service: $40 (or whatever you customarily charge for an exam and vaccination). Of course, we won't administer the vaccine without a physical exam.

What's different about this approach is the "packaging" of the service and the pricing strategy. Why would a client pay $10 for a service that his or her trusted veterinarian provides for free?

If the particular month you select for the promotion doesn't correlate with the local ordinance, simply give the client a certificate entitling him or her to the free vaccination when it's due.

Among the benefits of this program:

- The offer creates value for the client. We save the client some money on the rabies vaccination (a required service), and give him or her comfort regarding the pet's wellness (an optional service).

- We're practicing defensive marketing. The people who take advantage of this offer won't be lured away by the vaccination clinic; plus, they're more likely to comply with the ancillary services we recommend.

- We get to see these clients and patients at least once more than we would have otherwise. And, because it's a slow time of year, we'll be able to spend more time on each animal—increasing our ability to identify and perform needed ancillary services.

- We'll spend less time on the animal when it returns for its vaccination because we recently performed a comprehensive exam. Therefore, we have the ability to see more patients during the busy season and/or to spend more time on the animals we haven't see recently. The end result is greater efficiency and additional opportunities to identify needed services.

- Most clients will return to receive the free vaccination, so we'll have an automatic call-back vehicle to emphasize compliance with recommended procedures.

- We'll collect fees months earlier than we would have otherwise, smoothing our cash flow.

The above strategy is only one example; others may include wellness plans, special seasonal pricing, an emphasis on compliance with non-critical services through aggressive call-backs (e.g., geriatrics, dentistry, behavior counseling, skin and coat care, or other wellness programs) or targeted data base marketing. Please note that an important goal of seasonal businesses is to push work from peak periods to off-peak periods. Spreading cash flow throughout the year helps everything from staff scheduling to paying the bills.

Just rewards

As we wrapped up our study, one thing was clear: Veterinarians deserve to do better. Making honest money through hard work and practicing good medicine is no crime; however, given your educational accomplishments, the long hours you work, and the capital you've invested in labor, facilities and equipment, the failure to make good money *is* a crime. If you don't like the "business" of veterinary practice, find a competent financial advisor to run your hospital for you.

Such an arrangement is known as "outsourcing," and it is becoming more popular every day. Or, bring in a competent hospital manager to take care of the business. Spending money will save you money *and* time. But whatever else you do, keep in mind that opportunities in veterinary practice abound—and that you deserve your just rewards.

Source:

Arthur Andersen and Co., P.O. Box 13406, 1500 Commerce Tower, Kansas City, MO 64199-3406; phone (816) 221-4200.

This article originally appeared as "Outsiders spot problems, opportunities in practice" in the November 1993 issue of *Veterinary Economics*. It is reprinted here by permission of the publisher.

Proactive pricing

by Ross D. Clark, DVM

Proactive pricing is the single most effective management tool you can use to cause an immediate and dramatic increase in your net income.

During February, typically the lowest grossing month of the year in most parts of the United States, many of us are probably wondering what we can do to improve our financial picture in the coming year and how we will pay our taxes and first quarter tax deposits come April 15th. In order to find solutions to these problems, I have attended a number of conferences on fee setting and pricing. This part of the chapter covers some of the most exciting points brought out at those conferences.

Dr. Meir Karlinsky of Carnegie-Mellon University said, "Fee structure and pricing can be as easy as you want it to be. It can be simple, quick and ... *wrong*!! Good pricing, on the other hand, is the result of a synergetic combination of rigorous art and creative science used to decide rationally on issues which involve a lot of irrationality." Good pricing, in other words, is proactive.

And proactive pricing is *not* basing your fees and price on cost. Veterinarians from time immemorial have been looking for the perfect pricing based on cost. Pricing based on cost is not only very difficult; it is not always competitive and effective in today's world. Consumers base their buying decisions on perceived relative value, not on the providers' costs.

What proactive pricing *is*:

The concept of proactive pricing can be summed up with these two statements:

- Be a price-maker, not a price-taker.
- It is fair to charge what the traffic will bear on some items in order to make up for areas of your business where

profit margins are necessarily narrow or in which you actually are losing money.

What is involved here is the difference between the contemporary concept of verum pretium (natural prices) and the ancient concept of justum pretium (fair prices.) Natural price is reached by agreement between willing buyers and willing sellers. Fair price is one in which the seller adds only as much to his buying price (cost) as is customarily sufficient for his economic support, with no unfair enrichment. Veterinarians want to charge a fair price. However, in the marketplace a fair price can be too high and chase clients away.

Fair pricing is based on the medieval Christian view of how an economy should operate justly. The word "fair" stems from "fagar," an Old High German word meaning "beautiful." Can we make a price (a mere number) more fair? More beautiful? Findings and theories from behavioral decision theory, which deals with the framing of decisions for problems, suggest that indeed we can.

Almost all American companies make small profits in some areas while reaping huge profits in others. According to pricing authorities, the total cost of ingredients in a bottle of America's leading pain reliever is seven cents; yet this bottle sells for $2.99.

Built in along the way is plenty of room for advertising, shipping, and a huge profit margin. Veterinarians need to move toward this model to compete in the contemporary marketplace.

As veterinarians, we have a concept of being fair that says, "Give me a fair markup on some of the things that I do, and I'll conduct the rest of my business for cost or less for educational purposes and/or goodwill." The reaction we have to unfair price is, in part, the result of our fuzzy and impressionable evaluation of the value of the item. Any information about its low cost affects our perception of its worth, and we hesitate to charge more than what we believe to be its worth. We must begin to think of "worth" in other terms. An item may be "worth only

$1.00." Our "worth" or expertise in using this $1.00 item may consist of many years' "worth" of experience and education.

Guidelines for setting proactive price structures

1. *Consider your variables.*

Price structure is the set of product and purchase characteristics along which price levels vary.

Examples:

Typical Taxicab Price Structure (based on cost):

- Price to get into the cab

- Price per mile

- Price per minute

Alternative Taxicab Price Structure (based on value):

- Flat fare by zone

- Price per passenger

- Premium for telephone usage

- Premium for peak hours

Pricing based on value is the method by which most organizations conduct business. If veterinarians insist on fair markup across all services and product lines, then some services and products will be considered too expensive by some clients and you will lose market share.

In addition, the remaining services and products may not generate enough income to keep the clinic profitable.

2. *Don't lower your prices (without careful analysis).*

Be aware that every one-percent decrease in price requires a four-percent increase in volume to net the same profit. If a one-percent decrease in price requires four percent more volume, then a 10-percent decrease in price requires 40 percent more volume to net the same profit. Therefore, always be *very, very, very careful* before you even consider lowering the price of a product or service. Lower prices can only be justified if it will generate a significant increase in sales, enough increase in fact to increase profits. Don't forget that when you lower the price on an item or service, that lower price is not confined to the additional products or services sold, it also applies to the products or services you could have sold for the original higher price.

3. Appeal to various market segments.

Market segmentation develops price structures that offer different prices for different market segments. Market segmentation attempts to attract the price-sensitive, bargain-seeking customer while retaining the full-price, full-service consumer. Examples include hotels with their seasonal rates, weekend rates, corporate rates and better-than-corporate rates; airlines with first-class fares, business-class fares, nonrefundable fares, tourist-class fares, coach-class fares, 30-days-before-flight super-saver fares and frequent-flyer bonuses; and gas stations with full-service prices, self-service prices and discounts for cash.

Example in airline price structure:

Problem—Want to increase tourist volume without foregoing business customer revenue.

Differentiating factor—Tourists generally spend weekends at destination; business customers do not.

Solution—Offer discount fares for itineraries that include a Saturday night stay.

Examples in veterinary medicine price structure:

Problem—Want to increase the volume of price-shopped services without foregoing current customers who desire full service and are willing to pay full price.

Differentiating Factor—Most clients are more concerned about convenience than with price and want full service, so they will come in for regular office visits more often.

Solution—Offer a half-price Veterinary Technician Vaccination Clinic one or more afternoons a week that does not include a doctor's exam. If the client wants a doctor's exam, he or she must step to another exam room and pay an exam fee. This will appeal to clients more concerned about price alone.

Problem—Want to appeal to price shoppers in general.

Differentiating Factor—Many price shoppers are senior citizens that have the time and motivation to price shop.

Solution—Offer senior citizen discounts to clients over the age of 65 on weekdays between 1 and 4 p.m. Rather than lower prices on basic services, try to add value by offering additional services or products when basic services are purchased. Such additional services might include:

a) "Go-home" injections for pain at check-out time*
b) Safety and comfort packages with surgeries and dental procedures*
c) Fluoride treatments with spays/neuters
d) Tattoos or microchip placement at the time of spay/neuter*
e) Nail trims ("pedicures") with surgical procedures
f) Dental prophylaxis with surgical procedures
g) Frequent buyer food discount
h) Food delivery service one day a week

*See Practice Workbook, "Surgical/Medical Forms"

Summary

Veterinarians must begin to build the cost of their "worth" into their practice structures. The more "cutting edge" services and technology you offer the more "worth" you need to build into your pricing program.

Clients are smart ... if your clinic is clean, progressive, convenient and customer-oriented they know they "get what they pay for." There will always be those who refuse to acknowledge or understand that progress is expensive and that a knowledgeable staff is as important to the well-being of patients as a doctor who subscribes to continuing education.

There are people who should not have animals, who begrudge spending a dime on an animal. Sometimes you and your staff can win them over with patience and marketing. Sometimes nothing works.

Do not set your price structure for these latter people. You can't please them. Rather structure your prices for those who know high quality costs more and who are aware of the "worth" of your services.

Chapter 2:
Human Resources

Careful hiring and extensive training

by Ross D. Clark, DVM, and Jan Coody, MBA, Hospital Administrator at Woodland PetCare Centers

If you are tired of personnel problems, start your practice turnaround with careful hiring and extensive training. Successful business firms have recognized for years that a high turnover of employees is expensive and counterproductive. Everyone should recognize that good employees are a veterinary hospital's most valuable asset.

However, when a vacancy opens, there may be a tendency to hire the first person who walks through the door, particularly if you're in the midst of a hectic day. Be forewarned—most employee problems start at this point, by hiring the wrong person. Most of these problems can be eliminated by making a concerted effort to hire more carefully.

Don't let an employee's approaching departure date intimidate you into a rushed decision with too few choices. Take the time and get enough candidates to make a quality decision. Hire a temporary assistant if you have to. In the long run, you will have less stress, lower training costs and less turnover. Here's how to maximize your chances of hiring a winner.

Everyone should recognize that good employees are a veterinary hospital's most valuable asset.

Things to do:

Maintain a file of drop-in applicants: These people have revealed both self-motivation and a specific interest in veterinary medicine. If they qualify, they have the potential of becoming happy employees who remain with your organization.

Recruit from technology schools: These students have shown their self-discipline by taking the proper steps to prepare for a career in veterinary medicine.

Advertise: Word your ads carefully and include as much information as possible (e.g., location, hours, salary range, type of work, and other requirements) so as to limit time-wasting phone calls from inappropriate applicants:

> ***Location.*** By listing the general location of your hospital, you won't be troubled by applicants who live too far away.

> ***Hours.*** If you are looking for an employee for only Saturdays or evenings, clearly stating the part-time nature of the job will save the applicants' and your time by producing only applicants looking for those hours. For

part-time help to cover evenings and weekends, run ads in local high school and college newspapers. For part-time adult help, consider using classifieds in the local "ad-sheet" tabloids.

Salary. By listing the salary range, you will not need to read resumés and interview scores of well-qualified applicants who are unwilling to work for the usual veterinary employee's salary. Make the salary competitive; you get what you pay for.

Type of work. For positions of ward attendants and maintenance personnel, ask the applicants to apply in person.

Requirements. If your practice needs a receptionist or an exam room technician, ask applicants to submit a resumé and a handwritten essay in 500 words or less about why they want the job and why they are best qualified.

When relatives, friends and clients show an interest in working at your hospital, hand them the same application form and ask them to submit a resumé and a handwritten essay. Treat them as you would any applicant. File the applications along with those responding to your help wanted ad, and invite only the most qualified people for interviews. Caution: Don't let your personal feelings about your relatives, friends and clients cloud your judgment. Ask yourself if you could discipline a friend or Aunt Sally's daughter if the need arose.

Applications and interviewing

Forms: Have all applicants complete a detailed application form that includes a list of references. Application forms that meet all equal-opportunity legal requirements can be obtained from your local supplier of office products.

Interviews: Always conduct an extended interview (usually 20 to 30 minutes). Keep the resumé and application in front of you as you ask questions. If you're hiring a receptionist, make it a point to speak with the applicant on the telephone to hear how he or she will sound to your clients.

Be sure to ask the following questions in your interview:

- "How do you feel about humane euthanasia?"
- "Would there be any objection to working weekends or evenings?"
- "Do you have transportation to and from the job?" (You'll be surprised at how many applicants fail to figure this out before accepting a position.)

- "Tell me about your early life and other job experiences." Be an active listener, but allow the interviewee to talk for at least 60 percent of the time.

Tests: Be thorough in your interview by administering appropriate skill tests. I recommend asking potential receptionists to rearrange 50 random patient cards into alphabetical order and file them. Check carefully for accuracy. (See *Practice Workbook*, Section 4: Staff Search Forms, for a sample pre-employment test.)

Tour: Give each candidate a tour of the hospital. This step allows you to observe the applicant's interaction with other employees as well as with the patients in the hospital. Since about 60 percent of our communication occurs through body language, it is important to observe the applicant's body language during the tour and interview process.

Observations and evaluations: Get some feel for loyalty and honesty from what you learn about the candidate's lifestyle. He or she should like animals, but not be obsessed with them. Note the applicant's attention to detail and neatness on the application form. Note also his or her apparent health. At our practice we look for employees who are, above all, friendly. A new employee will need to get along with veterinarians, coworkers and clients in order to do the best job of marketing and delivering our services. For the same reasons, flexibility is equally important.

***Job description*:** Be sure to bring a written hospital policy manual and a thorough job description to the interview. Discuss these documents with the applicant and listen to the person's reactions. (See *Practice Workbook*, Section 6: Job Descriptions.)

***Reference checking*:** Check references by telephone rather than by letter. Previous employers will be more candid on the phone because there's no written record of their comments for which they may later be drawn into court if the job candidate feels he or she has been maligned. Ignore written references brought to you by the candidate. Letters by former employers are often written out of guilt. Sometimes they are written by the candidate themselves. Check with most of the former employers about the candidate. The most recent employer may not have negative things to say, but the previous one may have had problems you would like to hear about.

Some key questions to ask are:

- "What can you tell me about the applicant?"
- "Can you comment on professional strengths and limitations?"
- "Would you hire this person again?"

Don't overlook this important step of checking references. It takes time, but it's essential. In my consulting, I often find that an employee problem could have been avoided had references been properly checked.

Hiring

Notification: After you have made your selection, call the winning applicant first, to be sure that person is still available for the position. Then call those interviewees whom you did not choose and tell them they were highly qualified but that you've chosen someone else. Give good reasons to help preserve the applicant's self-esteem. For instance, say that the person selected had seven years of experience as a receptionist in a small-animal hospital in Denver and was familiar with the type of computer you plan to install soon. Don't say that someone was smarter or seemed to have a more outgoing personality than another. Strive for good relations. Remember, the person you turn down may be a future client.

Negotiation (salary and incentives): A good rule to follow: Pay the right price for the right person, within reason. It is nearly impossible, however, for owners of veterinary hospitals to compete with giant corporations when it comes to salaries and tangible fringe benefits. Therefore, we need to consider incentives other than salaries that veterinary offices can offer.

Incentives: Learning why the applicant wants to work for you will help you determine what will keep that person happy (and employed by you).

Schedule: In today's world, with nearly everyone in the household working, many employees are looking for a flexible schedule. Some want to be home when the kids get home from school, while other people want to escape their daily grind at home with the kids and spend more time with adults.

Personal satisfaction: Some want to work with animals no matter what the salary is.

Experience: Still others are young and would work for you simply to obtain job experience and possible continuing-education opportunities.

First things first

Begin cautiously: Always hire a new employee for an introductory period. Emphasize that you will be reviewing the worker's progress from time to time and that at the end of the introductory period (usually 30 to 90 days), you will meet and discuss the potential for more permanent employment. If you elect not to hire the applicant at that time, you may not be liable for unemployment compensation. Also, inclusion in group insurance policies can be postponed until the applicant gains the status of a permanent employee. Ask new employees to wear a trainee badge during this period. This will let the new employee and your hospital off the hook should minor errors in communication occur with clients. If the new employee does not work out, be firm and let him or her go. Don't stall. The longer you wait, the more painful it will be for all concerned, and the problems will multiply.

Assign buddies: Starting on Day One, assign a buddy who is familiar with the new employee's position to review the job description and to take the new employee around the hospital for introductions.

Clarify job description: After his buddy has introduced him to his coworkers and reviewed his job description, let your new worker view an orientation film. Ask him to review this film once a day for a week, and then once a week for six weeks. During the training period, use clear, concise descriptions of what you expect.

As examples:

> "We will expect you to greet clients with a smile." "You'll need to get the client's name, telephone number, address and method of payment before he or she is taken to the examination room."

Remind them to review the job description very carefully.

Get feedback: It's usually a good idea for someone from management to take the new employee to lunch on this first day and review any questions that may have developed during the morning. Remember to get feedback. Ask the employee, for instance, to repeat your instructions to be sure you've made them clear. Establish a completion date for the projects you assign, fill out a two-part memo, give the original to your staff member, then file a copy in a jobs-in-progress file box. Then follow up.

All things in time

Hold meetings: It's a good idea to include all of your employees in a general staff meeting at least four times a year. In addition, you should meet every two or three months with members of each department in the hospital to get their input.

Offer continuing education: It is also a good idea to include your assistants in professional seminars as much as possible. It does, in fact, improve their skills, and it demonstrates your interest in them and recharges their batteries so they can return to your practice with new skills and renewed inspiration to do a better job.

Conduct reviews: After hiring, orientation and training, you'll need to follow up with a periodic review every three months the first year and yearly thereafter. Do not combine reviews with salary increases. If you do so, the employees will only be listening for the last 45 seconds.

All of the above may seem like a lot of effort just to hire and start a single employee, but experienced personnel managers will agree that your time and money will be well spent.

General concepts of personnel management

by Ross D. Clark, DVM

"When the best leaders' work is done, the people say,
'we did it ourselves.'"

Lao Tzu, Chinese philosopher

The old industrial model many veterinarians follow puts the people who deliver services (receptionists, technicians and ward attendants) last. The new model puts front-line people first and designs business systems around them. The old model felt it was better to depend on technology rather than on human beings. The old model asked little of potential employees. As veterinarians, we used minimal selection criteria (often merely the ability to show up on time) and set only average to below-average performance expectations. We wanted to pay minimum wages and expected little more in return.

But a recent article in *Harvard Business Review* notes:

The more technology becomes a standard of delivered services, the more important personal interactions are in satisfying customers and in differentiating competitors.

The new model for practice management values investments in people. The contemporary practice manager must make recruitment and training as crucial for receptionists, technicians and kennel personnel as it is for veterinarians. Modern management links compensation to performance.

Hire the right person

A good interview technique is to describe a situation or task and ask the prospective employee what action he or she has taken in similar situations and what results he or she experienced.

To measure service attitude: "Tell me about a time when you went above and beyond the call of duty in serving a customer. What was the situation and what did you do? What was the result?"

To evaluate persuasion ability: "Tell me about a time when you were trying to persuade someone to do something and they resisted. What did you do? What was the result?"

To evaluate the applicant's moxie under stress: "I know I sometimes get uptight when I have to deal with an irate customer. Tell me about a specific experience you've had dealing with a difficult customer. How did you handle it? What was the end result?" (For more interview questions, see the *Practice Workbook*, Section 4: Staff Search Forms.)

To attract and keep motivated employees:

- Make the application a little more difficult and be more careful with hiring procedures.

- Interview each final prospect at least four times.

- Always have an introductory period.

- Train with the "buddy" system.

- Motivate by delegating responsibility and giving positive reinforcement when a job is done well. Give a lot of "mental fringe benefits."

- Remember: Things that get rewarded, get done; things that get measured, get done.

- Keep a more harmonious office by having at least four staff meetings a year.

Yogi Berra is sometimes quoted, "If you don't know where you're going, you will probably end up someplace else." For employees to have a strong sense of direction, it is always important that your clinic or hospital have a mission/vision statement of purpose that:

- Sets a clear direction;
- Reminds employees why they come to work;
- Establishes operational priorities;
- Provides a vision of the future;
- Builds a sense of proprietorship; and
- Appeals to a higher purpose.

Vision is like a link between dream and action. A vision must capture people's hearts. Without a goal, neither companies nor people get anywhere.

Vision is like a link between dream and action. A vision must capture people's hearts. Without a goal, neither companies nor people get anywhere.

Frequent hiring mistakes

Hiring mistake #1
Failure to check references by phone. Failure to ask, "Would you hire this person again?"

Hiring mistake #2
Selecting the applicant with the highest qualifications rather than the applicant with the best matched qualifications.

Hiring mistake #3
Failure to have an introductory period (formerly known as a probation period).

Hiring mistake #4

Failure to use skill tests and other measures of mental acuity. An intelligent employee, regardless of level of education, will usually be less prone to make mistakes and will, therefore, be happier in the job.

Firing

If you do make a hiring mistake, I recommend that you approach firing in the following manner:

- Implement the firing process by giving employees a clear written warning of their job (not personal) deficiencies. Initiate suggestions on training available to help the employee with his or her problems.

- Follow up with two additional written warnings. On the third warning, suggest that the employee doesn't appear to be very happy in this job (if that seems to be true) and that you are prepared to give him or her three days off with pay to find other jobs that might be a better fit.

- Tell them that you have no choice but to let them go. Do not delay firing too long. As Dr. George Burch of Pitman Moore once said, "It takes a dairy farmer two years to sell a kicking cow and a veterinarian two years to fire a bad receptionist."

Codicil: If you have an "at-will" hiring and firing policy in your employee manual and your state laws allow you to have such a statement, you may terminate employment for any reason at any time.

Things to remember when hiring and firing

- Familiarize yourself with legal issues regarding hiring. Dr. Jim Wilson's book, *Law and Ethics of the Veterinary Profession* (Yardley: Priority Press, 1988), is a good source.

- Focus on attitudes rather than qualifications. For example, you might say, "Tell me about a work experience in which you weren't treated as you wanted to be."

- Conduct multiple interviews:

    a) One interview by the hospital manager or owner

    b) One interview by the staff with whom the prospect will be working

    c) A follow-up interview for the top three or four applicants by both the hospital manager and staff members.

- Find the right fit. Management guru Brian Tracy says, "When you hire someone, you're just trying to find the right fit between the job and the person." When you explain this goal to applicants, it helps them relax because they realize you aren't judging their personal worth.

- Always check references. It's important to ask the applicant's former employer, "Would you re-hire this person for the same job?" Make "peer to peer" calls. If references are from a veterinarian, a veterinarian should call. If references are from an office manager, an office manager should call.

- Start with a trial period. Ninety days is typical. In most states you can decide not to hire someone during this 90-day introductory period with no repercussions. Also, there is no requirement for employers to provide benefits, such as health insurance, during this period—as long as you treat all new hires alike.

- Realize that benefits are important to some people. Salary may be less important than you think. Some people can't manage their money, so rather than take home a larger sum to pay for their own benefits, they'd prefer more benefits as part of their compensation package. When tailoring these packages, however, be aware of state and federal laws regarding benefit packages as a tax deduction. These laws are constantly changing.

- Search for employees in the off season. Good employees work all around us, and you should keep your eyes open for prospective staff members. We assume, incorrectly, that the wonderful receptionist at the bank wouldn't want to work for us. You'll never know unless you ask. If nothing else, she'll appreciate the compliment.

Codicil: "You can make more friends in two months by becoming interested in other people than you can in two years by trying to get other people interested in you." Dale Carnegie.

Source:

Brockmeier, J. "Hire the right people the first time, 'de-hire' them if you have to." *Veterinary Economics.* June 1991: 62-63.

Streamlining the review process

by Thomas G. Diffell, DVM

"She hasn't been here a year already, has she?" I asked myself, staring at the technician's personnel file.

"Okay," I sighed, *"I'll review her next Wednesday, right after surgery. Let's see, how much of a raise did I give the last technician at her review? I'll just give this employee the same thing; better to keep fair. I think I did that other technician's review last month—or was it the month before? I sure wish I had something written down. This is the last thing I have time for right now."*

Sound familiar? As the busy owner of a small-animal practice that employs four full-time technicians, one full-time and two part-time kennel attendants and a part-time receptionist, I used to postpone employee reviews until the last minute. Why? Because I didn't think I did them very well. But a few years ago I decided to improve the way I handle this important but dreaded practice-management responsibility.

The first step: February reviews

My staff is important to me and to the practice's overall performance. They deserve to know what behavior I value and expect. They also need to know how I will evaluate and compensate them for their performance. Although I found an employee manual tremendously helpful in communicating such information, it wasn't enough. I needed a consistent, relatively painless method of evaluating my employees.

For me, trying to keep track of every employee's hiring anniversary had proved to be disastrously difficult; so I decided to review all employees the first week in February regardless of when they had started. January is typically a slow month for me, so I knew I would be able to devote that time to preparing their reviews.

I implemented the new schedule by counting the first February after an employee's initial three-month review as the start of his or her evaluation cycle. For example, if a technician starts in June, his or her three-month review takes place in September, but the regular annual review begins the following February. Even if he or she starts in December, the initial review takes place in March and, again, the first annual review would take place the following February.

> *Although I found an employee manual tremendously helpful in communicating such information, it wasn't enough. I needed a consistent, relatively painless method of evaluating my employees.*

The first three months

I consider the first three months of employment a training period. Every new employee receives a written job description and a list of tasks for which he or she will be responsible. I assign a staff member to monitor the employee's progress; at the end of the three-month training period, I meet with the trainer and ask if the new employee has mastered his or her assigned responsibilities. I also want to know how well he or she handles instruction and correction; what kind of attitude he or she displays toward clients, patients and coworkers; and whether the new employee behaves as if he or she likes the job.

Then I meet with the new employee to discuss the trainer's observations and to allow him or her to talk about the job. I may give a small raise. At this time, full-time employees may apply for health insurance and they become eligible for one day off without pay per month of service, to a maximum of five days, until the following February.

The annual review

At the end of January, each employee signs up for a 30-minute appointment during which I will go over a written review (see *Practice Workbook*, Section 8: Personnel Review Forms"). To make my life easier, I've set up a review form on my computer which allows me to type in the appropriate responses each year. I also refer to the employee's last review to remind myself of our previous discussion. In addition to the employee's name and title, start date, date of last review, starting salary and current salary, the form includes the following sections:

- *Strengths.* Here I list five to 10 of the employee's primary strengths, which may include promptness, good phone skills, excellent venipuncture technique, an ability to take criticism and so on. I discuss each strength with the employee in detail.

- *Improvements.* Here I note improvements made in any areas discussed during the previous review. For example, an employee may now be better at reading differentials, using the computer, dealing with clients and so on.

- *Weaknesses.* No matter how many weaknesses an employee may exhibit, I limit the list to the two or three worst, using specific examples whenever possible. I might note, "Needs to improve bladder catheterization of female dogs," or "Needs to be more patient with new staff members." I make sure the employee understands each weakness; we then discuss how to correct the problems.

- *Goals.* For each listed weakness, I provide specific steps the employee can take to overcome it. For example, if a technician is having trouble catheterizing female dogs, I may ask him or her to practice by passing a catheter through a euthanized dog, with a proficient technician's help. I also list any new responsibilities I want the employee to handle. I've found, for example, that giving a new task to an employee who gets impatient with new staff members can help the employee become more understanding of the pressures new employees face.

- ***Compensation package.*** Under this heading I list all forms of compensation the employee receives, including such benefits as uniforms, free pet care, vacation time, sick time, continuing education and insurance. Next to most of the benefits, I simply write "as per manual" because our benefits are based on length of employment and job title; the employee's hourly wage, however, depends solely on his or her skills, strengths, improvements and weaknesses. Before the meeting, I print one copy of the review form for the employee and one for his or her personnel file. Both the employee and I sign each form.

Year-round monitoring

To ensure that I accurately evaluate my employees' performance and attitude *throughout* the year, I keep a work-performance file for each employee in the computer. I document such patterns as arriving late for work, missing veins or behaving rudely to clients or coworkers. I also note each time I see an employee "going the extra mile" and every occasion on which a client compliments a staff member.

Recording such examples of on-the-job behavior takes only a few minutes, and it allows me to refer to specific strengths and weaknesses during the review. I adjust compensation only during the annual review, but I meet with my employees more than once a year. If I detect a consistent problem or find that an employee is doing an outstanding job, I address the situation immediately.

Consistency and peace of mind

My review process brings consistency to what was once haphazard, but there are other benefits as well. Now employees can see how far they've come and note the relationship between higher pay and increased skills and responsibilities. Outlining their total compensation package also reminds them that the practice provides more than just their hourly wages.

This review process is so successful, in fact, that one year I reviewed my entire staff during a two-hour car trip on a get-away weekend with my wife. She drove, realizing that I wouldn't have to work late throughout the trip—or the year—to pull together last-minute reviews.

But, best of all, I no longer have to ask myself, *"Oh no, is it that time again?"*

This article originally appeared as "She's been here a year? Dusting off your employee-review process" in the July 1994 issue of *Veterinary Economics*. It is reprinted here by permission of the publisher.

Winning staff meetings

by W. Bradford Swift, DVM

Your favorite basketball team is playing its arch rival. At the end of the first half, the buzzer sounds and the two teams run off the court. As you watch from the stands, the coach and his assistant stroll over to the timekeeper while your team circles around the water cooler. In a few minutes, the referee blows his whistle and the two teams walk back to center court.

You think to yourself, "What, no locker room pep talk? Not even a huddle? What's going on?" You glance at the scoreboard to confirm that your team is behind by six points. How can they expect to come back in the second half and win the game without coaching?

You can't win if you don't coach

Now think about your own "game" in veterinary practice. When was the last time you "coached your team?" If you're wondering why you're coming up short each month on your scoreboard, why employees circulate through your practice like a revolving door or why your staff is always complaining, maybe it's time to call a time-out—with a staff meeting.

I know what you're thinking. For many of you, staff meetings simply don't live up to your expectations. In working with hundreds of small business owners and other professionals, I've found that for most, staff meetings are difficult to schedule, disorganized, time-consuming and unproductive. That's why many people, including veterinarians, don't schedule them anymore. And even those who do schedule staff meetings often find that employees arrive in body, but not in spirit.

What would you say, however, if I told you that staff meetings could increase your practice growth by 15 to 20 percent, or more? And what if each meeting inspired you and your staff, and gave you an action plan for making the next month extraordinary? Would you give them another try?

One more time

In my early years of practice ownership, I hated staff meetings. For starters, they were impossible to schedule. When I did manage to schedule one, it was a disaster. They were so bad, I finally stopped scheduling them—and no one complained. It took me years before I had the courage to try again. When I did, I got an unexpected surprise. With help from a management consultant and plenty of trial and error, I began to learn how to lead powerful and effective meetings that improved the quality of my practice. I entered these meetings with four distinct goals:

- *Clear the air.* In the course of running a busy practice, tempers flare, cross words are spoken, arguments are started and feelings get hurt. Left unresolved, such matters can eat the heart out of the most successful team and even cause valuable employees to leave. Staff meetings give everyone an opportunity to resolve conflicts *before* a blow-up occurs.

- *Acknowledge and appreciate team players.* In a busy practice, employees' contributions often go unrecognized. Regular staff meetings are perfect opportunities to acknowledge hard work both individually and collectively. Complimenting an employee publicly can be an effective tool for inspiring his or her best performance. It also helps to smooth employee relations when staff members acknowledge each other. Remember, no contribution is too insignificant to be recognized.

- *Check the score.* Sometimes it's tough to look at the scoreboard during the game. Calling a staff meeting gives everyone a chance to catch their breath and check the score. Is the team on track? Are you winning the game—or falling short? Staff meetings also allow employees to evaluate their own performances and to make sure the results are in line with the practice's goals.

- *Adjust the game plan.* Staff meetings give you the opportunity to coach your players. Perhaps your team has strayed from the game plan or you need to adjust your strategy. It's better to know where you stand at half-time than after the final buzzer.

Where to begin

Effective staff meetings begin with a commitment to producing them. Before we could hold such meetings in my practice, I had to understand that all of the bad meetings in the past didn't mean future ones had to follow suit. I listened when other veterinarians told me how important staff meetings were to their practices. I began to realize that just as I could never spay a dog without being trained, I couldn't expect to lead effective meetings without learning that skill. Here are some of the strategies I learned that worked particularly well:

- *Identify the purpose of the meeting.* In one or two sentences, summarize what objectives you intend to accomplish. Doing so gives the meeting focus and helps keep everyone on track.

- *Plan ahead.* Never walk into a meeting without specifics on what you want to accomplish, what issues need to be discussed and who needs to attend. Provide a copy of the agenda prior to the meeting so that the participants have time to prepare. Another point to consider: Unnecessary staff meetings only make the important ones more difficult, so make sure a meeting is the best way to achieve your stated purpose. Talking with one employee or sending a memo may be all that's necessary to achieve the desired result.

- ***Start and end on time.*** Establish a clear time frame for the meeting and stick to it. Employees hate coming to a meeting on time only to wait 15 minutes for latecomers, or attending a meeting that runs over by 30 minutes. Stress the importance of being on time to everyone invited.

- ***Involve others.*** One of the biggest obstacles to an effective meeting is a leader who tries to do everything: Lead the meeting, record the minutes and make sure the meeting stays on track. I've found that meetings are more effective when these tasks are delegated to a three-person team.

- ***End with a specific action plan.*** Reserve the last quarter to one-third of the meeting for developing an action plan. Such a plan specifies what actions need to be taken, who will take them, and when the actions should be completed. This step alone turned my staff meetings into productive, powerful sessions.

- ***Decide when and with whom to have meetings.*** Every practice has its own schedule and set of circumstances, so it's up to you to decide the best time for meetings. As you plan, keep in mind that successful meetings start with a commitment. If you commit to one full staff meeting a month for the next six months and apply the principles I've outlined, I think you'll find that the meetings aren't as difficult to schedule as you might have imagined.

You also may determine that not every employee needs to attend every meeting. For example, if the purpose of a meeting is to increase the number of annual check-ups and routine vaccinations, you may need to meet only with your front-office personnel. If the meeting includes the entire staff, consider holding it outside the hospital after hours. To build team spirit, you may want to include dinner or a time for socializing before the meeting. Such occasions can be well worth the time and money invested.

Meetings can make a difference

In my practice, I went from avoiding staff meetings at all costs to scheduling them on a regular basis—and looking forward to them. In fact, when we started meeting every morning for 15 or 20 minutes to be sure everyone was ready to play their best, my practice became more enjoyable and productive than it had ever been. It still wasn't always easy to find the time for staff meetings, but we noticed the adverse effects when we slacked off.

Staff meetings gave my team the opportunity to rally when we were slipping—just like a basketball team that's down at the half and emerges from the locker room to come back and win the game. Now *that's* a powerful meeting.

This article originally appeared as "Coach your team with winning staff meetings (Part 3)" in the November 1993 issue of *Veterinary Economics*. It is reprinted here by permission of the publisher.

Staff training and review

by Ross D. Clark, DVM

"The main problem with American companies is their failure to train."
Ross Perot

Few situations are as frustrating for your staff as not knowing how to do their jobs properly or what you expect from them. Far too many veterinarians hire new employees, tell them how welcome they are, then turn them loose. Even if a new employee has experience, he or she isn't familiar with the unique ways your practice conducts its business.

As an untrained employee's stress and embarrassment grows, your workplace becomes uncomfortable for everyone, including your clients. Not only do you stand to lose a potentially valuable employee, you may begin to lose clients. Staff training and review are critical components of practice renewal and success.

To avoid either outcome, I suggest you take steps now to implement stringent hiring procedures and an in-depth training program in your practice. No matter how great we may be as clinicians and managers, few of us can handle every situation that arises. That's why a well-informed, well-trained staff is critical to a healthy and successful practice.

Four steps to a training strategy that works:

Develop job descriptions. Every position in your hospital, from kennel technician to intern, should have a written job description listing the specific duties to be performed.

Assign a mentor. Every new employee should be assigned to a senior staff member who makes sure the new person understands what his or her job entails and helps the newcomer perform his or her duties in a timely and professional manner.

Sample training checklists appear in the *Practice Workbook,* Section 5: Staff Training Materials.

Produce a training video. Every practice should have a training video for its receptionists, cashiers, and exam-room and kennel technicians. These employees work in plainly visible areas, so systematic procedures are important. For example, orders should be opened and closed the same way every time. Clients should never get the impression from a cashier that the fee for a particular service might vary or that there might be a mistake in the bill. And each client should be served in a timely manner that doesn't make him or her feel rushed or afraid to ask questions. Also keep in mind that the more comfortable your receptionist and cashier feel using your hospital computer (or whatever system you use), the more competent they will appear to your clients.

Producing a training video can be a hospital project that occurs over the course of several evenings. With your own video camera, or perhaps one borrowed from a staff member, videotape your head receptionist demonstrating the system your hospital uses. Your cashier can do the same thing for his or her position. After you've edited the tapes, they will become invaluable training tools.

Cross-train your employees. Your employees should be thoroughly trained not only to perform their own jobs, but to know the jobs of other employees as well. Cross-training effectively ensures that you have sufficient paraprofessionals and support staff available at all times, particularly if your hospital offers extended hours. Cross-training also can help your budget by allowing you to employ more part-time employees and cut back on the number of full-timers. Most important, cross-training makes all of your employees valuable members of the team, which is much better than relying on a few indispensable people.

Empower staff

With an effective training program in place, your next step is to empower your employees to take advantage of their unique talents. Keep in mind that power builds confidence; and happy, confident employees mean happy, loyal clients. A few suggestions:

- *Encourage team spirit.* Regularly remind your staff that you are a team, and that no employee is on his or her own.

- *Follow the Golden Rule.* Treat each employee as you would like to be treated.

- *Follow the Platinum Rule.* Treat each employee as they would like to be treated.

- *Encourage suggestions.* A suggestion box is still one of the most effective ways to get feedback. Be sure to implement some of your staff's ideas. If their ideas work, your staff will develop the confidence to suggest even better ways to serve clients and save time and money. If you feel strongly that an idea won't work, be prepared to explain why. Remember, it takes a certain amount of risk to promote growth.

- *Share information.* It's important to share your goals with the members of your staff and listen when they share theirs. For example, post hospital goals in the employee lounge each month. Post your practice's gross revenue each day as compared with last year, as well as your goal for the current year. Should you meet these goals, be sure to thank staff members with bonuses and/or a celebration.

Trust staff

In the long run, it's a waste of money to train and empower your staff if you don't trust them. You can demonstrate your confidence by encouraging employees to:

- *Educate clients.* Your staff members frequently spend more time with clients than you do and, thus, have more opportunities to educate them. Clients, who sometimes fail to listen to you because they're asking questions while you're talking, may be more receptive to your staff.

- *Find out what your clients really want.* Many clients fail to tell the veterinarian what they want from him or her and are not fully satisfied when they leave. A friendly staff member with a confident, professional approach often can head off a potential problem.

- *Keep the best interests of your practice at heart.* If you train your staff well and empower them to make decisions for the benefit of the team, your hospital's goals will soon become their goals.

Turn up the heat

If staff problems don't convince you of the importance of implementing a serious training program in your practice, competition from large pet superstores with excellent training programs just might. These superstores are not only intent on offering your clients low-cost spays, neuters, vaccinations, pet-care products and toys—they plan to offer "Gold Star" service!

In this age of self-service, more and more clients are looking to over-the-counter medications and vaccines to stretch their budget; and these large, corporate-owned stores may fill the void. They may become to small-animal medicine what Wal-Mart and K-mart have become to small-town hardware stores, and what giant grocery store chains have become to locally owned pharmacies.

To compete with these powerful superstores, satisfied clients are no longer enough. We need loyal clients. One of the best ways to inspire loyalty in our clients is to employ a team of professional, highly trained, front-line people who are committed to customer service and client satisfaction. They are our best chance for success.

What staff members say about owners

by Carin A. Smith, DVM

As a relief veterinarian, I've found that I'm a convenient "sounding board" for disgruntled employees. Although it's human nature to complain about your job once in a while, I've discovered that in certain hospitals, more than the usual amount of staff complaining occurs—and many employees are quietly looking for another job.

The comments in this article are a compilation of the most common complaints I've heard during six years of relief work. You may not know it, but here's what your employees are saying about *you*:

Who's doing what?

"I wish we had job descriptions," one receptionist told me. "I was hired to work at the front desk, but when it gets busy in back, I'm often called to help. But I'm not trained to do that kind of work, so I end up feeling frustrated. Meanwhile, clients are kept waiting in front, and the phone doesn't get answered as quickly as it should. We could see far more patients if we had a second technician to absorb some of the work and allow me to do my job."

At another hospital, a technician told me he feels limited by the work he *isn't* allowed to do: "I haven't done any lab work since school," he complained. "My knowledge is going to waste. I'd like to learn more, but the doctor won't give me time off to attend continuing-education classes. I think he's afraid that I'll try to 'play doctor' with the clients, but I only want to do what I'm trained to do."

Such complaints provide clear evidence that when employees don't understand—or agree with—their specific duties, frustration and resentment result. The lack of clear direction from their employers also seems to give some employees license *not* to take responsibility. For example, I asked a receptionist at one hospital where I might find a specific type of flea shampoo, but instead of looking for it herself, she replied, "You'll have to ask Debbie."

I soon learned that only Debbie could answer most of my questions. The other employees weren't new on the job—it was just easier and faster to "ask Debbie." Heavy reliance on one person is easy to overlook because such dependency builds gradually. But remember: when "Debbie" eventually quits from exhaustion, she'll leave a chaotic hospital behind.

Inter-staff conflicts

My experience shows me that disagreement over hiring procedures is another tension builder in many practices. "Our hospital just hired our third receptionist this year," one employee complained. "We end up with people who have never held a desk job in their lives. The most recent receptionist had never even owned a pet! I think it's a good idea for the staff to be involved in the hiring process, but the boss needs to provide some minimum standards as well."

A receptionist at another practice explained her frustration with new hires this way: "The doctor won't let any of her staff have input on new employees. She hires people with impressive qualifications but who lack the people skills necessary to gain the clients' respect. Our new technician scared off several of our clients because of the way he handled their pets. But the doctor trusts him so much she doesn't even monitor what's happening."

Practice owners who hire family members present another potential problem for employees. Although such employers vow that they can separate their personal and professional lives when they hire a son to be a kennel worker or a spouse to be a bookkeeper, here's an example of what their employees say: "If I have a problem with any other employee, I can talk to the boss about it. But not when it comes to our accountant. After all, who's going to complain about the doctor's husband directly to her? I'd lose my job if I did."

Other complaints are similar: "We all get along with the doctor's wife on a personal level," one employee said, "but sometimes she changes roles in the middle of a conversation. I can't tell whether I'm speaking to the bookkeeper, the office manager or the spouse. Sometimes she and the doctor give me conflicting instructions, and I don't know whose orders to follow. Everyone else has a job description, and I wish she did, too."

Other veterinarians unknowingly present situations their staff finds intolerable. For example, at one hospital, the owner set aside an extra room where her kids could play after school without interfering with hospital business. Unfortunately, the arrangement backfired for the staff: "We can't get anything done when her kids are around," the receptionist said. "The doctor thinks it's cute that her kids are learning to help, but they're in the way. They interrupt us constantly, and even bother clients—who don't think the kids are as cute as the doctor does!"

So much to do, so little time

"We're sorry to see you go," a technician once told me. "It's been so organized while you were here. Doctor Joe won't come in until after 9 a.m. tomorrow, and by then, the clients will be backed up in the waiting room. The in-hospital treatments won't be done until noon! Then we'll end up working past 6 p.m. just to get caught up."

Dedicated practice owners often forget that time off is important to their staff. Although your employees share your concern for patients, you should realize that they will never be as committed to their jobs as you are. You can expect your employees to be flexible when necessary, but they won't tolerate long hours that are forced on them because of *your* work habits.

Appointment policies that interrupt the hospital's schedule may cause frustration as well. Many practices have a no-appointment policy and operate on a first-come, first-served basis, with emergencies taking priority. Although many practice owners believe that allowing clients to bring in their pets at a moment's notice is a necessary service, consider the effects that such a policy has on your staff:

"I'm the one who has to soothe all those frustrated people in the waiting room, and it's driving me crazy," one receptionist said. "Yesterday, Mrs. Jones was kept waiting for 45 minutes. She threatened to leave if she wasn't seen immediately, so I had to sneak her in ahead of someone else. And we lose a lot of clients who just can't wait."

Before you write off this employee's complaint as simply an unfortunate fact of practice life, consider her suggestions for improving the situation—which her boss isn't even aware of: "I have several ideas about how to improve our schedule," she said. "We could set aside certain days for walk-ins, and schedule appointments on the remaining days. But the doctor never asks my opinion, and I don't think he perceives a problem."

Fair wages, fair charges

You may be surprised to learn that the biggest complaint I hear during my relief assignments does *not* have to do with salaries and benefits. Nevertheless, employees do feel frustrated when they see financial inequities. For example, some practice owners plead lack of funds when it's time for pay raises, but their employees often see where the real problems lie: "I was supposed to have my annual review two months ago," a technician said. "I'm overdue for a raise, but the boss keeps putting it off, saying he can't afford it. Yet he hasn't increased his fees for three years. Why should I suffer because he undervalues and undercharges for his services?"

At another practice, fees aren't the problem—the division of revenue is: "Our hospital policy includes the goal of prosperity for all staff members," an employee said. "But the only person I see getting prosperous is the boss. She's increased her fees every three months for the past two years, but we haven't even gotten a cost-of-living raise this year."

Your hospital's payment policies may be another area where employees see unfairness: "We have a cash-payment policy, but it seems as if the rules are bent every day," said a receptionist. "The doctor often interrupts me while I'm in the middle of trying to collect payment to tell me to let that person charge. And he gives reduced prices without any system I can see. I'm put in the position of being the 'bad guy,' and our clients know they can manipulate the boss to get what they want."

Legitimate gripes?

By now, you may be thinking to yourself, "Who's running this show? It's my hospital, and I'll run it as I choose. If I give in to every little complaint, the staff will be running me! Besides, my hospital is functioning smoothly—what's the problem?" The problem may be that you aren't listening to your employees—or to their legitimate concerns. But remember, satisfied clients depend on a cheerful staff eager to serve their needs.

When your employees are distracted and upset by other concerns, they suffer—and so do your clients. Should you listen to every little gripe, though? In other words, how much complaining is "normal"—and when does it reflect a real problem? You can bet that when all of your employees voice the same complaint, it's legitimate. Instead of blaming your staff for being unable to accept the realities of their jobs, however, you should realize that there may be room for improvement in the way *you* run your practice.

Resolving staff complaints has the added benefit of reducing employee turnover, saving you time and money because you won't have to repeatedly interview, hire and train new employees. Plus, your clients will be reassured when they're greeted by a familiar face behind the reception desk, and hear their calls answered by a staff member who remembers them and their pets.

Tell them to speak up!

If employees are so frustrated, why don't they voice their concerns and offer constructive criticism to the boss? One technician, who's worked at a hospital for five years, explained her reasoning for keeping quiet this way: "Talk to the boss? You've got to be kidding. If I spoke up, I'd lose my job. The doctor does a great job of studying practice management, but it's clear that she doesn't really want to hear what we think. I'm looking for another job, but I don't want to lose this one yet."

Another employee offered this defense: "We used to say what we thought at our monthly staff meeting, but it became clear that our boss was a good listener and nothing more. Changes that we suggested never happened, and worse, we often suffered for bringing up an issue."

How *can* you encourage your employees to speak up? First of all, your staff must know that you consider their job satisfaction a top priority. No amount of staff meetings can take the place of genuine concern and respect. Your employees will work harder if they feel that they, and their work, *truly* matter to you.

First of all, your staff must know that you consider their job satisfaction a top priority. No amount of staff meetings can take the place of genuine concern and respect.

To tap into employees' true feelings, provide a way for them to make anonymous suggestions, and arrange for occasional private discussions, in addition to regular staff meetings. Make it clear that you will not only listen but will incorporate their ideas when appropriate. If you don't agree with an employee's proposal, be sure to explain your reasoning so that he or she understands your decision. Most important, whenever your employees submit great ideas, thank them for their suggestions—then use them.

The best way to demonstrate that you care about your staff's input is to follow through on your promises and adhere to the policies and fees you establish. And when employees must enforce your policies, support them; when you respect your employees, they'll return the favor. Best of all, everyone will enjoy coming to work, client satisfaction will improve—and so will your bottom line.

This article originally appeared as "What are your employees saying behind your back?" in the February 1993 issue of *Veterinary Economics*. It is reprinted here by permission of the author and the publisher. In addition to practicing veterinary medicine, Dr. Smith is the author of "The Relief Veterinarian's Manual," "The Employer's Guide to Hiring Part-time and Relief DVMs" and "101 Training Tips for Your Cat."

Ten ways to boost morale

by Ross D. Clark, DVM

A college professor, after finishing a long speech on better methods of farming, then asked the farmers present if there was anything else they would like to know. One farmer raised his hand and said, "Professor, I don't believe so, because we've already been knowing more than we've been a doing." In the area of employee morale, most veterinarians already are "knowing more than they are a doing."

Employee morale is a common problem in today's business world. *U.S. News and World Report* estimates that 25 percent of U.S. workers—24 million people—are unhappy in their jobs, with resultant loss to their employers of billions of dollars yearly in poor workmanship, reduced productivity and absenteeism.

Morale is difficult to measure, but most managers agree that satisfied workers produce more. Morale in an organization does not mean simply that people get along well with one another. The real test is performance. If high morale can result in increased performance, then it is worth cultivating. If low morale is eating away at your organization like a low-grade infection, why not try some or all of these 10 steps to build a new sense of cohesiveness among employees as well as higher job satisfaction and increased production?

1. *Give praise when it's deserved.* When employees do a good job, tell them. Sounds simple, but it is surprising how many veterinarians neglect this elementary measure. Blanchard and Johnson's well-known book, *The One Minute Manager*, offers these suggestions:

- Tell people up front you are going to let them know how they're doing.

- Praise people immediately.

- Tell people what they did right.

- Tell people how good you feel about what they did right, and how it helps the organization and the other people who work there.

- Stop for a moment of silence to let them "feel" how good you feel.

- Encourage them to do more of the same.

- Shake hands or touch people in a way that makes it clear that you support their success in the organization.

2. *Delegate authority.* Few things can be worse for morale than a veterinarian who refuses to delegate authority. Those guilty of this common mistake seem to be saying they do not trust subordinates to make the right decision or to do a good job. A substantial role in the decision-making process, on the other hand, can boost morale appreciably. Studies show that workers given increased responsibility exhibit greater job satisfaction and produce more. Veterinarians should look at their willingness to delegate.

3. *Encourage the establishment of specific goals.* Many management authorities feel that this can be one of the most effective morale-building factors, particularly in group situations. Marks and Spencer, a British chain retailer, is one of the most successful companies of its kind in the world. A key to its success is its highly developed system of performance goals and standards, which are converted into work assignments that every employee can understand. Psychologist Jan Berkhout says that high-morale groups are always associated with tangible goals. He compares work situations with military and athletic endeavors, in which goals seen as attainable and worthwhile help to create high morale.

4. *Clarify expectations.* What is it you really want of your employees? While every supervisor can probably answer this question with ease, many workers might find it more difficult to say just what they think management expects. Confusion over the expectations of supervisors is one of the chief causes of worker dissatisfaction. Workers need to be told exactly what they are expected to achieve and, if necessary, where they are falling short. Vagueness, on the positive or negative side, is of no use to anyone. One effective tool is a standardized system of employee evaluations. The Japanese have long stressed formal, regular evaluations of worker performances. While many managers shy away from one-on-one evaluation sessions out of awkwardness or stress, this kind of communication can dispel confusion and bolster morale. An effective evaluation system need not be rigid or complicated; but it should be administered uniformly to all personnel and it should identify employee strengths as well as areas needing improvement.

5. *Keep employees informed.* Tell employees about upcoming events, policies and conditions affecting them. The complaint, "I never know what's going on around here," can be an anathema to a healthy working atmosphere. "Employees need to feel involved in everything," says Richard Corrada, director of personnel at King's Dominion, an amusement complex in Virginia. Corrada advocates frequent meetings at every level of organization. Other communications include employee newsletters, production progress reports and well-maintained bulletin boards. Employees need to be informed not just about policy changes, but of the reasons for them.

6. *Encourage worker feedback.* Communication is a two-way street; workers' ideas should be heard and considered. One way to accomplish this is through many staff meetings. Employees who feel they are part of the decision-making process are more likely to be satisfied workers. In the Federal Republic of Germany, employees of most companies play a direct role in corporate affairs. Through membership in councils protecting workers' rights as well as in actual representation on governing boards, they routinely participate in the management process.

One of the most substantial benefits of participatory management is its dampening effect on rumors. Through frequent discussion of substantive matters, gossip-mill misinformation can be corrected early.

7. *Adjust environmental and scheduling factors.* Improving the workers' physical environment can be an effective morale booster. Physical surroundings have a direct bearing on job satisfaction. Privacy, roominess and noise level are significant factors. Performance levels are higher for clerical personnel in quieter, roomier work spaces.

Similarly, allowing employees flexibility in work schedules can be highly effective. The use of "flextime" has become increasingly common in Switzerland, other European countries, the United States, Canada and Australia. Under this system, employees choose work schedules which suit their individual needs, often helping combat absenteeism in the process.

8. *Be realistic in counting on material rewards.* It is a common misconception that workers who are paid well exhibit high morale. While money can be a basic source of motivation, management experts have long recognized that social and psychological needs are in many ways more important. As long ago as the 1920s, work such as that conducted at Western Electric Company began to emphasize social and organizational factors in motivation. Many studies, most notably those of famed psychologist Abraham Maslow, show salary to be a relatively insignificant job satisfier. This does not mean that good wages and benefits are not necessary, but they must be kept in perspective.

9. *Fight boredom by providing change.* Take advantage of what Peters and Waterman, authors of the best-selling *In Search of Excellence*, describe as the "Hawthorne effect:"

In the late 1930s on the shop floors of Western Electric's Hawthorne plant, Elton Mayo of Harvard tried to demonstrate that better work-place hygiene would have a direct and positive effect on worker productivity. So he turned up the lights. Productivity went up, as predicted. Then, as he routinely turned his attention to another factor, he routinely turned the lights back down. Productivity went up again! For us, the very important message of the research that these actions spawned, and a theme we shall turn to repeatedly in the book, is this: It is attention to employees, not work conditions per se, that has the dominant impact on productivity (many of our best companies, one friend observed, seem to reduce management to merely creating an endless stream of Hawthorne effects) (Peters and Waterman).

10. *Be morale conscious.* New approaches to employee job satisfaction are constantly being developed. The wise manager will keep tabs on recent developments and be creative in applying them.

All things considered, the most important element in building and maintaining high morale is concern for worker satisfaction, combined with a communicative approach on every level of management. Nothing beats direct, creative attention on a day-to-day basis.

Sources:

Blanchard, K., and S. Johnson. *The One Minute Manager.* New York: William Morrow, 1982.

Peters, T., and R. Waterman. *In Search of Excellence.* New York: Harper & Row, 1982.

Rowh, M. "Building a happy workplace." *Rotary Magazine.* Chicago: Rotary International, 1982.

Developing an equitable incentive program

by Will Novak, DVM, MBA

Christmas was always an exciting time at the clinic and not just because of the Christmas party. There were also the annual bonus checks and pay raises to look forward to.

Stacey had been with the clinic for two years and had received a modest bonus along with a pay increase the previous year. That gave cause to hope for better times ahead. She thought to herself, "I work as hard as anybody here and I am pleasant to people. I deserve a raise, at least, or a bonus." The bonus would be helpful with year-end bills.

As always, Dr. Owner went around quietly during the party, pressing a small envelope into each staff member's hand.

Stacey anxiously opened her envelope. She was anxious to see how big her bonus would be this year. All she found, however, was a Christmas card—no bonus, no pay increase and no explanation. "What," Stacey asked herself, "have I done wrong?"

Unfortunately many clinics' incentive programs for staff are based on informal procedures. This leaves the employee to guess what actions will be rewarded and how much the reward will be. And most employees, like Stacey, have no idea how their work performance translates into bonuses and pay raises or the absence of either.

To boost employee morale with an incentive program, you must understand employee needs. To have that improved morale benefit your clinic's bottom line, you need to have a clear idea of what employee behaviors your clinic needs to nurture. As Dr. Ross Clark, with Woodland PetCare Centers in Tulsa, observes, "people do what they get rewarded to do." To work effectively for your clinic, rewards have to be tied directly to the performance desired and they must relate to a mixture of intrinsic and extrinsic factors.

Intrinsic factors include praise, recognition, personal growth, autonomy and completing a project—factors that are internal and have no monetary value. Extrinsic factors—such as salary, commission, fringe benefits, bonuses, vacation days and promotions —possess external, material value. Some extrinsic motivators are practical for a veterinary clinic and others, such as promotions, are not. Most clinics do not have enough levels within the organization to allow a receptionist or technician to be promoted very far.

Much has been written on intrinsic factors and though it is an important aspect of overall employee satisfaction, it must be considered *with* extrinsic factors. Extrinsic factors, especially pay and bonuses, are the basis for compensation and need to be specifically and clearly implemented before intrinsic factors can be considered important to an employee. Intrinsic factors are not meaningful to an employee if extrinsic factors have not been addressed.

While veterinarians have commonly compensated staff members on an hourly basis in the past, today's competitive environment calls for pay-for-performance arrangements like those used in large corporations.

Pay incentives have three goals. The first is to recruit good people. The second, to motivate current employees to high job performance. And the third, to keep good employees from leaving. Each of these objectives requires a different mix of intrinsic and extrinsic factors for total employee job satisfaction. Some interesting points have been noted from research on how employees judge different pay systems:

Satisfaction with pay is based on how much employees consider they should receive versus what they actually receive. It is important to identify what an employee considers fair in relationship to what they are paid. Interviews with veterinary staff have shown that 46 percent say their compensation is "probably fair." Can you do more to increase your staff's perception of the fairness of your compensation system?

Amount of pay received influences what is judged as fair, based on what others in the same job receive. This certainly demonstrates that standardized incentive programs are important to employees. Informal policies and unequal treatment will always produce negative morale with staff.

People differ in what is important to them concerning pay and benefits. This point may seem obvious except that many clinics still adhere to a set package of pay and benefits for all staff. Why not offer flexible benefits if this helps to attract the best employees?

The following methods can improve employee morale and performance and decrease your turnover rate, while addressing the goals of pay incentive:

Skill-based pay

This system has been little used in veterinary medicine, but it deserves great attention. It is especially useful in motivating and keeping current employees. Skill-based pay creates a stair-step system that increases the salary or hourly wage based on the demonstration of skills. This is especially appropriate for technicians who have a great variation in skill levels when starting a job. Many times veterinarians start with untrained employees and teach them as they work. Some of these employees learn quickly; others never master certain skills.

Skill-based pay provides support for personal growth through pre-set goals, a sense of achievement from reaching new skill levels and financial rewards with higher pay. All of these address both intrinsic and extrinsic motivation factors. As an employer, you receive a highly skilled staff member with a set path for improvement. If the employee cannot or will not go beyond a set skill level, then no pay increase is warranted.

This system can be used with or without seniority or sales bonuses. To implement a skill-based pay system, it is necessary to outline what skills are mandated at each level. The list of skills can be tailored to your clinic's specific needs.

For example, a system might have four levels. The first level could cover skills such as basic animal care. The next level might include medication preparation and dosage. The next level could include certain laboratory tests; and the fourth, more advanced technical skills. Testing should be conducted before promotion to the next level. Research at two companies showed that workers compensated in this fashion displayed more motivation to develop job skills, were more satisfied with their pay, identified more closely with their jobs and found it easier to work within the company.

Cafeteria-style benefits

In this system, the employer sets up a list of options for the employee and sets a dollar limit on the total benefit package. Options might include medical coverage, vacation, retirement or cash benefits. This allows the employee to have an active role in choosing the benefits that have the greatest value to him or her. Additionally, the economic value of the benefits become apparent to participating employees, who might not have fully realized the financial value of their benefits. The cafeteria-style benefit program should be used with some other bonus pay system. The disadvantage to this incentive system is that it is more complicated to administer.

Individual and group bonus methods

A bonus method is commonly used in many veterinary clinics, generally with some salary base. I have seen it implemented on a group and an individual basis. The group method can have variations, for example, exceeding this month's gross revenues versus the same month last year. Some of these programs have very complex formulas, many times too detailed for the employee to understand. The theory of this system is to provide team building and individual productivity with a pay incentive. In discussions with employees concerning group bonuses, I have recorded mixed results. Some employees are motivated by these programs, but it is common to hear that they do not feel individual efforts are directly rewarded. For a group system to be effective, it must be simple, have achievable goals and be clearly understood by the staff.

The individual bonus method has been commonly recommended by Dr. Clark. Bonuses can be based on any number of factors: pet food sales, heartworm tests, flea product sales, etc. Each staff member may receive a percentage commission on the sales they make. This system's strength is high individual motivation, but it requires individual tracking of sales, which can be time consuming.

The motivated, enthusiastic, energetic staff member is usually the one paid to perform. These different pay incentives, whether used individually or in combination, can make a difference in the effectiveness of your staff.

This article originally appeared as "Avoid a Stalemate in the Employee Incentive Game" in the September 1995 issue of *Veterinary Forum*. It is reprinted here by permission of the publisher.

Creating self-directed "dream" teams

by Ross D. Clark, DVM

"We must continue to grow. We must continue to profit. We must continue to return profits to our team and to society."

Dr. Kayria
leading practitioner and management consultant
Tokyo, Japan

Says Jon R. Katzenbach in his book, *The Wisdom of Teams*:

"We believe that teams, real teams, not just groups that management calls 'teams,' should be the basic unit of performance for most organizations, regardless of size. In any situation requiring the real-time combination of multiple skills, experiences and judgments, a team inevitably gets better results than a collection of individuals operating within confined job roles and responsibilities."

Teams are more flexible than larger organizational groupings because they can be more quickly assembled, deployed, refocused and disbanded—usually in ways that enhance rather than disrupt more permanent structures and processes. Teams are more productive than groups that have no clear performance objectives, because their members are committed to deliver tangible performance results. Teams and performance are an unbeatable combination.

The Internal Revenue Service increased collections by 33 percent with half the staff and one third of the branch offices. IBM has reduced their quote turnaround time from seven days to one day, while preparing 10 times as many quotes. By fusing information technology with new ways of managing people, veterinary hospital managers should be able to achieve major reduction in processing cost and improve quality and service at the same time.

Few people today question that a new era has dawned in which such high levels of performance depend on being "customer driven," delivering "total quality," "continuously improving and innovating," "empowering the work force" and "partnering with suppliers and clients."

The same team dynamics that promote performance also support learning and behavioral change. Teams will play an increasingly essential part in first creating and then sustaining high-performance veterinary hospitals.

Change has always been a management challenge. But, until recently, when executives spoke of managing change, they referred to "normal" change—that is, new circumstances well within the scope of their existing management approaches. Many people, however, would agree that change today has taken on an entirely different meaning. While all managers continue to have to deal with "normal" change, more and more must also confront "major" change that requires a lot of people throughout the company—including those across the broad base of the organization—to become very good at behaviors and skills they are not very good at now. The days of viewing change as primarily concerned with strategic decisions and management reorganizations have vanished. Here's how Jack Welch, Lawrence Bossidy and Edward Hood describe the challenge facing General Electric in their 1990 letter to shareholders:

> Change is in the air. GE people today understand the pace of change, the need for speed, the absolute necessity of moving more quickly in everything we do ... From that pursuit of speed ... came our vision for the 1990s: a "boundaryless" company. Boundaryless is an uncommon word ... one that describes a whole set of behaviors we believe are necessary to achieve speed. In a boundaryless company, suppliers are not "outsiders."

Every effort of every man and woman in the company is focused on satisfying customers' needs. Internal functions begin to blur. Customer service? It's not somebody's job. It's everybody's job.

Leaders today cannot succeed without the participation and insights of people across the broad base of the organization. Together, top management and the people who look to them for leadership must first identify and learn critical new skills, values and behaviors; then work to institutionalize those behaviors to sustain high performance. We believe teams are essential to such objectives because they have always induced behavioral change as both an ingredient and by-product of team performance.

Several well-known phenomena explain why teams perform well. First, they bring together complementary skills and experiences that, by definition, exceed those of any individual on the team. This broader mix of skills and know-how enables teams to respond to multifaceted challenges like innovation, quality and customer service.

Second, in jointly developing clear goals and approaches, teams establish communications that support real-time problem-solving and initiative. Teams are flexible and responsive to changing events and demands. As a result, teams can adjust their approach to new information and challenges with greater speed, accuracy and effectiveness than can individuals caught in the web of larger organizational connections.

Third, teams provide a unique social dimension that enhances the economic and administrative aspects of work. Real teams do not develop until the people in them work hard to overcome barriers that stand in the way of collective performance. By surmounting such obstacles together, people on teams build trust and confidence in each other's capabilities. They also reinforce each other's intentions to pursue their team purpose above and beyond individual or functional agendas. Overcoming barriers to performance is how groups become teams. Both the meaning of work and the effort brought to bear upon it deepen, until team performance eventually becomes its own reward.

Finally, teams have more fun. This is not a trivial point, because the kind of fun they have is integral to their performance. The people on the teams we met consistently and without prompting emphasized the fun aspects of their work together. Of course this fun included parties, hoopla and celebrations. But any group of people can throw a good party.

What distinguishes the fun of teams is how it both sustains and is sustained by team performance. For example, we often see a more highly developed sense of humor on the job within the top-performing teams because it helps them deal with the pressures and intensity of high performance. And we inevitably hear that the deepest, most satisfying source of enjoyment comes from "having been part of something larger than myself."

Behavioral change also occurs more readily in the team context. Because of their collective commitment, teams are not as threatened by change as are individuals left to fend for themselves. And, because of their flexibility and willingness to enlarge their solution space, teams offer people more room for growth and change than do groups with more narrowly defined tasks associated with hierarchical job assignments. Finally, because of their focus on performance, teams motivate, challenge, reward and support individuals who are trying to change the way they do things.

As a result, in the kinds of broad-based change that organizations increasingly confront today, teams can help concentrate the direction and quality of top-down leadership, foster new behaviors and facilitate cross-functional activities. When teams work, they represent the best proven way to convert embryonic visions and values into consistent action patterns because they rely on people working together. They also are the most practical way to develop a shared sense of direction among people throughout an organization. Teams can make hierarchy responsive without weakening it, energize processes across organizational boundaries and bring multiple capabilities to bear on difficult issues.

In fact, most models of the "organizations of the future" that we have heard about—"networked," "clustered," "non-hierarchical," "horizontal" and so forth—are premised on teams surpassing individuals as the primary "performance unit" in the company. According to these predictions, when management seeks faster, better ways to best match resources to customer opportunity or competitive challenge, the critical building block will be at the team, not individual, level. This does not mean that either individual performance or accountability become unimportant. Rather, the challenge for management increasingly becomes that of balancing the roles of individuals and teams versus displacing or favoring one over the other. In addition, the individual's role and performance will become more a matter for teams, instead of hierarchies of managers, to exploit; that is, in many cases teams, not managers, will figure out what the individuals on those teams should be doing and how they are performing.

Employees are empowered if they:

- Get information about organizational performance.
- Are rewarded for contributing to organizational performance.
- Have the knowledge and skills to understand and contribute to organizational performance.
- Have the power to make decisions that influence organizational direction and performance.

Cost of performance-based teams

Empowerment will have increased costs because you need to invest more in the careful selection of "self-directed" team members. Empowerment will also have increased cost because you must train "self-directed" team members more extensively.

Source:

Katzenbach, J., and D. K. Smith. *Wisdom of Teams: Creating the High Performance Organization*. Cambridge: Harvard Business School Press, 1993: 15-19.

Developing highly committed, self-directed, teams

by Tom Carpenter, DVM, partner/owner of the Newport Animal Hospital in Costa Mesa, Calif.

As owners of practices, we expect nothing but the highest commitment from ourselves. We often unfairly expect the same level of commitment from our employees. We ask, "Why can't you follow my example and show 100-percent commitment to the hospital?" The answer to that question is painfully obvious. They don't own it.

If we want our staff to share the values of owners, then we need to first examine our own feelings of commitment to see how we can positively affect those of our staff.

Committed owners:

- focus on the whole business;
- design the systems in the hospital;
- take risks;
- possess short- and long-term goals;
- are results-oriented;
- are client-driven;
- focus on continuous improvement;
- make short-term sacrifices for long-term gain; and
- make decisions based on sound financial management.

But if you want an *employee* to act like an owner, he or she must be treated like one.

It is unreasonable to expect an employee to act with the same responsibility as an owner if he or she is not treated accordingly.

We must empower our employees if we are to receive the commitment that we desire. Kimball Fisher, a well-known expert on self-directed work teams, defines empowerment as a function of four variables:

- Authority
- Resources
- Information
- Accountability

We often have a tendency to fail to delegate *authority* by giving the impression that it can only come from us. We must learn to give up control over our employees and to give them the authority to act on their own. There is a learning curve in doing this. Mistakes will be made. Progress will be slow. Patience is truly a virtue. Remember, as people step out and take the risk to act on behalf of your business, they are out of their comfort zone. The only way to expand their comfort zone is to praise them as they step out. We must become champions of risk-taking.

Resources and *information* come through the training and technology we provide. This should be a line item on every budget.

Accountability also originates from us. If we lead by the example of our own accountability, others will follow. We must learn to focus on purpose or solutions rather than problems.

If you fail to provide any of these four variables at any time, you will fail to empower your staff. Let us examine all of the characteristics of owners and see what our staff requires to acquire them.

Focus on the whole business.

Employees cannot focus on the whole business unless they are well informed. Everyone must know the goals of the hospital as a business. To take this one step further, they should participate in forming these goals. As an example, if we have a goal to provide every client with exceptional service, everyone must be willing and able to step outside the boundaries of their own position to do this. The culture of the hospital must be, "I will do whatever it takes to provide exceptional service." We need to get away from the "It's not my job" syndrome.

Design the systems in the hospital.

Systems are the framework of our operation. They must be continually adapted to changes in our market. As leaders, we must direct the development of systems in which our work teams can operate. We must ask for and require our staff's input in this process. Focus must be on end results. How can we best achieve the goal of this system? This system will be owned by both you and your staff.

Their input is necessary for the system to work. As your staff learns to step outside the boundaries of their positions, you will also have the added advantage of fresh points of view on how a system may be improved. Encourage this, or it will never happen.

Take risks.

Most of us grew up in environments that discouraged risk-taking. Control-oriented leaders do not seek out people who are willing to take risks. Institutions such as schools, churches and athletic teams are all traditionally control-oriented. The only way to break out of this mold is to reward the risk-takers. Praise is the most valuable tool. We have all experienced the warm feeling of being praised for stepping out and acting on our own to solve a problem. It makes us want to do it again and again. Encourage this at all levels of your business. Your actions define how you will be viewed. If you say you want people to act on their own but you don't react, soon they will think you don't care.

Possess short- and long-term goals.

Goals have been our secret for too many years. Even if we shared them with our staff, the goals didn't seem real to them because they had no idea how those goals were formed. In high-commitment work environments, the goals are set by the team and kept in front of them at all times. The whole team can't be expected to buy into goals that they did not help form.

Be results-oriented.

Traditional managers claim that they are results-oriented but in fact act like they are after control, not results.

Our principles need to be centered around results because we are empowering our people to obtain them. We lose many of the talents of our employees if we try to control how we get from point A to point B. Initiative can only be fostered by encouragement. Demanding that it be done "my way" won't work. If we are constantly hovering over our assistants, our actions tell our staff not to use their own initiative.

Ask yourself, "If clients need to be served in a way that doesn't fit our system, do I want them to be told that we don't do that?" In this case, we can ensure this doesn't happen by letting go of our staff. Get out of their way.

Be client-driven.

Several years ago my partners and I made a conscious decision to be more committed to our customers. To allow our hospital to become client-driven, we had to provide everyone, owners included, with extensive service training.

A large amount of this came from outside sources. We used speakers, videotapes, books and outside seminars. I found that not only did our staff become more committed; I did as well.

Chapter 2: Human Resources ■

Resources and information proved to be a vital part of this commitment. Commitment is highly contagious; blind faith is not.

Ongoing commitment to our customers is an ever-changing process because we find that our customers' needs are changing. Part of this commitment involves asking the customers what they want. Our team is much more willing to change if the need is expressed by the customers. Everyone is responsible for listening to the customers.

Focus on continuous improvement.

The surest way to establish a culture of continuous improvement is to ask for and acknowledge the help of the entire staff. This can occur with formal changes in the system or informal changes on a daily basis. The most important means of encouragement is open communication. Formal communication comes in the form of frequent meetings. Informal communication, which is equally valuable, comes in the form of chatter in the course of work. We must be willing to accept and encourage change as leaders before we can expect the rest of our staff to do the same.

Make short-term sacrifices for long-term gain.

We must agree that as an organization we will make sacrifices today for the benefit of the business tomorrow. When we talk of these sacrifices, we aren't always speaking of financial sacrifices. Training, which is probably the biggest key to success, is largely a sacrifice of time and effort on the part of our staff.

No amount of money can ensure success if those being trained don't buy into the need for it. It is very important to celebrate the success brought about by sacrifices. Again, these celebrations don't always need to be formal. Recognition is a reward that we all crave. It is easy, inexpensive and painless—if we could only remember to use it.

Make decisions based on sound financial management.

Fifteen years ago, when I started my career as a veterinarian, it was unheard of for management to share financial information with staff. This is still a scary process for most of us. Yet how often have we seen conflict arise out of incorrect assumptions? When we were employees, didn't we think that our bosses reaped all the benefits from the business? We made an assumption based on speculation because we had no access to the facts. In that case, those facts were financial information. As leaders, we should expect that nothing has changed in this regard. Our staff will make the same assumptions if they lack information.

Sharing financial information is only half the equation. We must also train our staffs to interpret that information. As we share information, we find that we have much greater understanding and commitment to our plans for the business. Again, we cannot expect our staff to act like owners if they are not treated like owners. I have never met an owner who doesn't want to know and understand the financial information of the business.

Compensation

The final aspect of treating the staff as owners revolves around paying them as owners. This can be done in many ways, depending on the preference of the owner. Compensation should be based, at least in part, on the performance of the business. This can be based on sales or on any other financial aspect on which the owner would like to focus.

We re-designed compensation at my hospital, basing it, in part, on gross sales. We also felt, however, that to accomplish our goals, we needed to focus attention on employee cross-training. To accomplish this, we included skill level in the plan. The skill-based system provides incentives for all members of the staff to learn areas of service in which they were not initially trained. By doing this, it is easier and more efficient for us to be client-driven. All wages of all employees are based on this system. A similar system could be designed as a bonus pool in addition to normal salaries, however.

Designing a system based on skill levels would have been difficult had we not asked for and received the help of our staff. They constructed skill-level checklists that enumerated and described all skills required of each work team. We then asked the members of each team which tasks could be crossed-trained for staff members not on their team. To receive an increased share of the compensation pool, they must both cross-train and put their new skills to use.

The resulting cultural change involves much greater interaction between work teams than we had previously experienced. They now depend on each other for training; but their interaction goes much further than that. To have this system work, they must:

- Recognize the need for help in their own work team.
- Recognize the need for help in other work teams.
- Learn to ask for help as needed.
- Learn to respond and help as needed.
- Celebrate the progress and acknowledge the whole team every time it works.

In our hospital, we have found this to be a tremendous learning experience for everyone. It has been successful financially, but, more importantly, it has improved the work environment dramatically. We call it "The Employee Partnership Program." I am happy to say we are all living it, and this is what it looks like in practice:

Implementing the employee partnership program

All employees at our hospital are paid on a percentage of the practice's gross sales. Eighteen percent of gross sales are split among employees, excluding grooming employees.

Compensation is determined by a team effort. Everyone is responsible. Financial gain is based on efficiency and growth of the business. Employees share in the success they create.

Advantages to owners

- Set percentage of gross is paid to paraprofessional employees.
- Allows better financial stability. Limits liability.
- Better team effort.
- Allows more self-management of staff.
- Creates team atmosphere.

Disadvantages to owners

- Could limit profit as the business grows.
- Responsible for much greater staff training in business: marketing, sales, leadership, service excellence, total quality management and cross training.

Advantages to employees

- They share in the success they help create.
- They learn concepts of business that will help them in all parts of their lives.

- Working as a cohesive team will generate more job satisfaction.

- A "partnership" arrangement empowers them to earn a steady increase in their annual incomes in two ways:

    by increasing gross sales,

    through improving efficiency and productivity.

Disadvantages to employees

- Doing something new can be uncomfortable.

- If productivity and sales stay the same, they lose income.

- Short-term players may not be rewarded.

Items critical to success

Teamwork
Everyone becomes responsible for the clinic's operation. Everyone has to take responsibility for serving clients. Everyone must be responsible for helping each other be better team members.

Cross-training
Everyone must learn all positions to increase efficiency. Everyone has to be willing to teach all the tasks they know to make that possible.

Team effort
Everyone has to work together to improve the performance of mediocre employees. Every member of the team has to be willing to share their strengths and address his or her own weaknesses.

Hard choices
Management may have to release poor team performers. High-performance team members need to understand the necessity of making these choices.

Playing fair

It is critical that compensation be fairly distributed among employees. A distribution system that is perceived as unfair will destroy team morale and undermine the entire "partnership" arrangement.

Why 18 percent?

The regional mean for staff compensation is 19.6 percent of gross, including grooming. Some practices in 1993 devoted as much as 25 percent of gross to staff wages. That is not a tenable distribution of practice assets. It's not good for the business. It strains the practice's flexibility and deprives it of necessary operating capital.

Increased capital in the business allows investments which will further improve the practice. These investments, although made only by the owners, will benefit all employees.

Trying to keep staff compensation *under* 18 percent, at the other extreme, would undermine staff morale and interfere with the practice's commitment to service and quality.

A working formula:

I recommend multiplying each employees "hours worked" by his or her "skill level," and then paying the employee 18 percent of that figure.

This plan excludes the grooming department, which will be treated separately. Grooming sales are included in the gross sales.

Rating system

1. Training period

2. Well trained at one position

3. Partially cross-trained

4. Fully cross-trained

5. Management

Theory of shared compensation

Looking into the future of our hospital, we saw a lot of hard decisions ahead. Like any business, to be successful we needed:

1. Annual growth.

2. Adequate capital.

3. Good quality management and employees.

For most veterinary practices, the key to success is number three. Some hospitals may get lucky and achieve numbers one and two, at least for a time, but clearly no hospital can sustain success without quality management employees.

Without annual growth of sales and adequate capital in the business, we would not be flexible enough to survive changes in the business economy and would be unable to make investments necessary to improve our operation. To do that we had to assemble a work force that took personal responsibility for the growth and success of the hospital.

We wanted our staff to think, act and get paid like owners. Everyone's individual actions needed to contribute to a team effort to improve the business. Employees now share in a percentage of the income of the hospital. That is, employees *own* 18 percent of the gross income of the hospital. This means that as the gross income increases, the 18 percent that the employees own grows as well. It also means that the performance of individuals, as a part of this team, has a real effect on the income of everyone involved.

We had no doubt in our minds that for this hospital to continue to grow, we needed everyone to share an owner's responsibility. To make that team effort possible, we strove to increase everyone's knowledge of business practice and principles. We informed our employees of and involved our employees in every step of the conversion process to an "Employee Partnership Program." We also brought in outside experts who were made available to everyone. We explained to employees that:

> Running the financial end of a business is very involved. When budgeting expenses, the expenses are placed into categories. Some of the categories are fixed expenses that do not vary from month to month. These expenses are not readily controllable. The other expenses are "variable." These change from month to month and are controllable. Fixed expenses include rent and utilities. Variable expenses are employment costs, drugs and supplies.

> When all expenses are subtracted from the gross sales, the remaining dollars are net to the owners. At Newport Harbor, we have three owners who work full time and when looking at the income that goes to the owners we must consider that they are paid as doctors. After a reasonable salary is taken out, the remainder is net for their investment in the business.

> A bank, which would be the most conservative sort of investor, expects a 10 to 15 percent return on its investment. If a bank lends money to a business, they charge 10 to 15 percent to lend the money. The interest reflects the amount of risk in the investment. When a private party invests in a business, most business advisors recommend at least a 20 percent return on investment.

> Over the years, owners of this hospital have invested a tremendous amount of their own money to buy the hospital. They have also invested a lot of what would have been net income back into the hospital to allow growth.

> This has been done largely in the hiring and training of quality staff. This is now and has always been our most

important investment. This high-commitment program will allow the staff to become much more involved in management decisions such as hiring, firing and training.

Skill level evaluation

If you choose to implement an employee partnership program in your practice, one of the ways you can begin to involve your staff in "real-time" management decisions is to call on them to help you create a set of cross-training checklists. You'll use these checklists to determine at what point a person has learned the skills necessary to be credited with the ability to "cover" a skill set outside of his or her usual job responsibility, the point at which he or she is fully "cross-trained." The numerous job-related checklists included in the "Staff Training Materials (Section 5)," "Job Descriptions (Section 6)," "Staff Procedures (Section 7)" and "Personnel Review Forms (Section 8)" sections of the accompanying *Practice Workbook* can serve as starting points for those discussions.

After the cross-training has begun and you start to conduct skill level evaluations, you should keep the following in mind:

- Credit for a skill requires complete knowledge of the skill. For example, someone who can do a dipstick on a urinalysis but can't read the sediment should not get credit for urinalysis.

- Credit for the skill means it is being performed whenever needed. Knowledge to perform a skill but not doing it when needed does not benefit your clinic. For this system to work, cross-trained techs have to help out receptionists when the front desk gets busy, and cross-trained receptionists have to lend the techs a hand when that operation needs it.

Hopefully this is not confusing. The basic premise remains that we want to give credit to those who are willing and able to perform tasks in different areas of the hospital to increase the quality of our service.

Notes on our implementation

May

An all-hospital meeting was called to introduce the new compensation program. At this meeting we emphasized cross-training and cross-functional teams. We used the Covey leadership training books to provide strong direction for our management group. Managers met weekly to discuss the book *Seven Habits of Highly Effective People* (New York: Simon & Schuster, 1989). We used this as a format to approach hospital relationships. In retrospect, we needed to do a better job of explaining the theory of the system and how important each individual is to the system.

June

We started the new payment program. We stressed cross-training and cross-functioning as much as possible on a daily basis. Initially there was a lot of confusion, and sometimes conflict, as employees started to move from position to position. People had to learn when and how to ask for help. Teams had to learn how to provide help to other departments and how to use the help other teams offered. As we got busier with the summer, managers met less frequently. Not many questions came up at this point regarding how the system of compensation worked. We found it necessary to offer praise over and over and over during this phase. We used a compliments board as well as written memos to encourage our staff.

July

The use of cross-training and cross-functioning began to get past some of the hurdles we had experienced in June. Departments began to develop interdependency, which was encouraging. People noticed that they were receiving an increase in pay.

August through November

Meetings were infrequent during this period. Business was good. People continued to receive increased pay. Nobody asked any questions. I assumed everyone was comfortable. I found out later that people were concerned about what was going to happen in the slower months. If I had known, I could have given them some idea; but as you know, predictions about future business are difficult.

December through February

During this period, there were three pay periods in which employees received a decrease from what their base pay had been before the program started. These occurred in slow periods which included holidays when we had people on vacation. The staff took this very poorly. We responded poorly. I guess we all learn by experience. I felt that they still had received an increase up to this point, between seven and nine percent per employee since the beginning of the program. I figured they should be happy. *Wrong!*

Some of the strongest negative reactions came from our best and most loyal employees. There was still concern about what was to come. I began to try to make everyone understand that the decreased earnings were a short-term phenomenon, that, in the scope of a year in business, it was nothing to worry about. This I might add was coming from someone who used to worry about turning out the lights to reduce his overhead in the slower months.

March through August

Again, business was booming. Pay went up. Everyone should have been happy, *Right?* Well, maybe. But business was so good that we had outgrown our systems of service. Without the cross-training *and cross-functioning* we never would have made it through this period. Although everyone could clearly see the value of this concept, we had systems that weren't adequately serving our staff or our clients. Fortunately, we now started to realize that our poor communication was about to extinguish all of our efforts to this point. We met and reformed our mission with everyone in the hospital. Nothing was new in principle, we had just gotten sidetracked. As a group we decided we needed to spend more time in preparing ourselves to meet our goals.

One thing had become crystal clear: We all value the work environment as by far the most important thing to all of us.

As we move into our second winter with this highly committed, self-directed and empowered team, we face the following challenges:

- Remembering to constantly analyze and evaluate the systems in the hospital.

- Remembering to create and maintain a training program on quality assurance that allows continued improvement.

- Determining how to measure the quality of our service on a continual basis.

- Continuing to study methods for building better self-directed teams.

- Remembering that we are staffing and scheduling based on interdependent systems rather than viewing each department separately.

Chapter 3:
Financial and Strategic Planning

Financial planning

by Jan Coody, MBA, Hospital Administrator at Woodland PetCare Centers

Financial planning is an important aspect of the business operation since it provides a map for guiding, coordinating and controlling actions to achieve its objectives. The two key aspects of the financial planning process are cash planning and profit planning. Cash planning involves the preparation of the cash budget. Profit planning is done by means of pro forma financial statements, which show anticipated levels of profits, assets, liabilities and equity. These statements are not only for internal planning but are also routinely required by lenders.

The financial planning process begins with long-run or strategic financial plans that in turn guide the formulation of short-term plans and budgets.

Long-run financial plans are financial actions that cover periods ranging from two to 10 years. A five-year plan is the most common. Long-run plans consider proposed fixed-asset purchases, marketing and major sources of financing. They may also include termination of existing projects, any planned acquisitions and repayment or retirement of debts.

Short-run financial plans are financial actions that cover one- to two-year periods and include the practice's sales forecast and various forms of operating and financial data. These include the cash budget, the pro forma income statements and pro forma balance sheet.

Cash planning

The *cash budget* or forecast permits the firm to plan its short-term cash needs. Short-term investments can be planned if a cash surplus is expected; or, if shortages in cash are expected, financing can be arranged. The budget gives a view of the timing of the expected cash inflows and outflows over the time period. Veterinary practices typically have seasonal cash flow patterns, making it best to plan the cash budget on a monthly basis.

The sales forecast is the key element in the planning process. Generally, a combination of external and internal forecast data is used in making the final sales forecast. The internal data provides insight into sales expectations based on the practice's history and the external data takes into account general economic factors. The general format for the cash budget is presented in Table 1.

Table 1. Forecast of a cash budget for a typical $300,000 practice

	October	Last Quarter November	December
Total cash receipts	$ 24,000	$26,000	$25,000
Less: Total cash disbursements	25,000	18,000	20,000
Net cash flow	$(1,000)	$ 8,000	$ 5,000
Add: Beginning cash	500	(500)	7,500
Ending cash	$ (500)	$ 7,500	$12,500
Less: Minimum cash balance	2,000	2,000	2,000
Required total financing	$ (2,500)		
Excess cash balance		$ 5,500	$10,500

Cash receipts include all cash inflows such as cash sales, collections of accounts receivable and other cash receipts. Cash disbursements include all cash outlays in the period. The most common are cash purchases, payments of accounts payable, rent expense, wages and salaries, tax payments, fixed asset outlays and interest and principal payments on loans. Depreciation and other noncash items are not included in the cash budget. The net cash flow is found by subtracting the cash disbursements from cash receipts in each period.

By adding beginning cash to the net cash flow, the ending cash for each period is found. Finally, subtracting the desired minimum cash balance from ending cash yields the required total financing or the excess cash balance. If the ending cash is less than the minimum cash balance, financing is required. If the ending cash is greater than the minimum cash balance, excess cash is anticipated.

Profit planning

The profit-planning process focuses on the pro forma statements, which are projected income statements and balance sheets. They require an accounting for the revenues, costs, expenses, assets, liabilities and equity resulting from the anticipated level of operations. The most popular approach is based on the assumption that the financial relationship reflected in the past financial statements will not change in the coming period. The simplified approach uses financial statements for the preceding year and the sales forecast for the coming year.

Pro forma income statement: A simple method for preparing a pro forma income statement is to use the percent of sales method, which forecasts sales and then expresses the cost of goods sold, operating expenses and interest expenses as a percentage of the projected sales. An adjustment needs to be made for fixed costs. Otherwise, profits will be understated as the benefit received from fixed costs will not be received. An example of a pro forma income statement using the percent of sales method with fixed and variable expenses divided is presented in Table 2.

Table 2. Pro forma income statement for a Woodland PetCare Centers Satellite Hospital

Last Year		Pro Forma
Sales revenue	$302,235	$332,459
Less: Cost of goods sold		
Fixed cost	0	0
Variable cost	$ 67,554	$ 74,305
Gross profits	$234,681	$258,154
Less: Operating expenses		
Fixed expenses	$169,076	$169,076
Variable expense	$ 18,786	$ 20,664
Operating profits	$ 46,819	$ 68,414
Less: Interest expense	$ 1,037	$ 900
Net profits before taxes	$ 45,782	$ 67,514
Less: Taxes *	0	0
Net profits after taxes	$ 45,782	$ 67,514

Pro forma balance sheet: A simplified approach for preparing pro forma balance sheets is to use the judgmental approach. The value of certain balance sheet accounts are estimated while others are calculated. When this approach is applied, the external financing is used as a balancing or plug figure.

Evaluation of pro forma statements

It is difficult to forecast the many variables involved in pro forma statement preparation. The basic weaknesses lie in the assumption that the past financial condition is an accurate indicator of its future and the assumption that the values of certain variables such as cash, accounts receivable and inventories can be forced to take on certain desired values. Even though these assumptions are questionable, this approach is quite common and widely used.

* Depends on form of business: corporation, partnership, sole proprietorship.

Pro forma statements provide a basis for analyzing in advance the level of profitability and overall financial performance in the coming year. The sources and uses of funds can be analyzed as well as various aspects of performance—liquidity, activity, debt and profitability. Various ratios can be calculated from the pro forma income statement and balance sheet to evaluate performance. Pro forma statements are therefore of key importance in solidifying financial plans for the coming year.

Source:

Gitman L. J. *Basic Managerial Finance*. New York: Harper and Row, 1989.

Strategic planning

by Brad Coody, MBA, accountant in Tulsa, Okla.

Vision

Who are you? What do you believe you can uniquely offer that the marketplace wants to buy? Work your vision into a mission statement that fits your core beliefs. From the mission statement, create a realistic set of attainable goals. This is critical because you never stray from your guiding principles. Understand them and work them into your action plans.

Work your beliefs into a system of what I choose to call permanent flexibility, which allows you to change and utilize new ideas and technologies yet maintain the integrity of your core beliefs.

Communicate your vision to associates who can share it, implement it and utilize it as a base on which to expand and grow. This interaction is, in my opinion, one of the key tenets to success in any field. (See also Chapter 6: How to work with banks and credit bureaus, "Writing a winning business plan.")

Selecting outside professionals

If you turn to outside professionals to assist you in your strategic planning, shop for accountants, lawyers, bankers, consultants and other professionals who have the time and talent to understand the unique nature of the veterinary practice. This does not mean selecting someone who is the most or least expensive. The selection process should include extensive interviews with each candidate. After all, you are hiring the professional for his or her ability to assist you in implementing your vision.

Seek professionals who can understand your objectives. You as a veterinarian should be able to learn from professionals the fundamentals of their disciplines without seeking a degree in each field. In short, seek professional specialists who will listen to your ideas, evaluate them and develop effective, workable solutions for you.

Strategic planning

As a veterinarian, you are most comfortable when you are one-on-one with a client. However, a successful practice involves breaking out of this "comfort zone" and developing action plans or strategies that will attain the results outlined in your mission statement.

Strategic plans should encompass broad objectives that direct the organization toward a level of attainable excellence. These plans are developed by defining broad guidelines that empower the practice's professionals and staff to practice in an environment that stimulates confidence while delivering quality service to the client.

Strategic plans should seek to provide a system of guidance while fostering creativity from the entire veterinary team. This is difficult for managing professionals to grasp at times; but, in my view, critical for sustained growth.

Security: Strategic plans should not be made available to the general public. Broadcasting your strategy can allow competitors to devise counter-strategies that could negate your unique advantage. In addition, announced goals can create untenable pressure on the staff if the goals are unrealistic. If it is your policy to publish a mission statement that is distributed to clients or potential clients, it is best to keep the statement general. In this way, you provide a level of flexibility necessary to consider new opportunities as they become available.

Cohesion: By keeping goals general, cohesion among peers and staff can be enhanced. It is much easier to support general statements such as "continued growth," "quality product" or "equal opportunity." These broad objectives can sometimes prevent serious rifts among the staff by focusing on those areas where there is substantial agreement. This approach treats more specific goal issues as decisions about concrete proposals or pro-gram details. It also focuses specific creative energies on solving goal conflicts in a logical and productive manner.

Quantification of strategic plans

In an ideal world, all activity would be quantifiable and measur-able. It is much easier to make decisions when quantifiable standards can be established to specifically measure a result. However, many strategic plans require decisions based on what customer attitudes and required service levels will be three to five years from now. Setting goals to ensure that personnel are motivated and trained to take advantage of new technological breakthroughs is not readily quantifiable. Thus, strategic goals must be defined and monitored effectively to avoid wasting resources.

Strategic planning requires leadership from senior management and an ongoing commitment to provide an environment that takes full advantage of the unique creativity of each staff professional.

Source:

Quin, J. B. Strategic goals: Process and politics. *Sloan Management Review*. Fall 1977: 21-37.

How to stimulate positive cash flow

by Ross D. Clark, DVM

Working *Capital* (spelled with an *"a" ...* the same as in *Principal*) is the lifeblood of your practice. It's hard to come by and hard to keep.

Where, outside of a bank loan, can you find the elusive "working capital" (aka cash)? Here are some of the methods I have known veterinarians, including myself, to use over the years, to acquire, manage and protect working capital. Some of these methods are quite expensive and must be weighed against the value or the consequences of not raising the needed cash.

1. Private investors or family members

This is usually the least expensive of all the methods. You may need to make the investor a silent partner or a partner depending upon the laws and practice act of your state regarding nonveterinarian ownership of veterinary practices. By the way, older successful practitioners in your state may be honored and happy to assist younger start-up veterinarians. Don't be afraid to offer them a piece of your practice in return for their help. Sometimes accounting firms will help companies find private investors for a fee of two to five percent of the money being raised.

2. Get tough with accounts receivable

When business is slow, ask your receptionist or office manager to call late, or non-paying, customers. Ask her also to forward the largest and toughest accounts to you for your personal attention. Clients are more likely to pay once they know their wonderful veterinarian is aware of their past-due account.

Minimize number of "days sales outstanding:" To keep your finger on the pulse of your accounts receivable calculate your "days sales outstanding" by dividing your monthly sales by the number of working days in the month. Then, divide your total accounts receivable by the average daily sales figure. Anything over 15 days is excessive.

Shorten the billing cycle: I do not know of a law requiring us to bill at the end of the month. One veterinarian I know moves the billing cycle back three days each month. At the end of 10 months, he has added a full billing cycle. Some critics question the value of this procedure because you would be adding the cost of postage and other billing expenses; however, if you are expecting a short fall, nothing prevents you from moving your accounts receivable to the middle of the month.

Convert accounts receivable to "Health Credit Cards:" At publication time there are four financial institutions offering credit to clients/patients of doctors, dentists and veterinarians. The following list is excerpted from an article published in AAHA's Trends magazine (December 1994/January 1995).

Care Credit
1-800-300-3046

- Four state dental associations endorse.

- To date ... veterinarian's clients charge about $197 per transaction.

- Clients spend about $550 on the first charge.

- AAHA entered into an agreement in November 1994 for discounted sign-up fee for members. Discount rate is five percent.

COMPLETECARE
1-800-879-2669

- Two types of accounts:

  —Funded for clients with a good credit history.
  —Post-funded for clients with a marginal, bad or non-existent credit history.

- Reports an average transaction of $125 to 150.

MEDCASH
1-800-800-5810

- Functions in a way similar to any MasterCard or Visa program.

- Has the lowest client approval rate of these four.

DENT-A-MED
1-800-262-3368
Similar to Complete-Care—two levels of accounts:

- Applicants with an excellent credit rating receive Gold account status. You pay a 4.5-percent discount rate and receive immediate payment from DENT-A-MED.

- Applicants with a marginal or bad credit rating receive Silver account status. You pay an 8.5-percent discount rate, plus a 16.5-percent charge that is placed in a bad debt reserve pool. You receive 75-percent immediate payment (versus 100 percent for good credit risks).

Ultimately it's a matter of choice for each hospital—and for your clients!

Leverage your accounts receivable: You can tap into your equity in accounts receivable by borrowing against those accounts receivable that are less than 90 days old or by selling your receivables outright—a process known as factoring. Lenders will usually loan you up to 80 percent of the value of non-delin-quent accounts. Factoring companies actually buy your non-delinquent accounts receivable at a discount of five to 15 percent, depending on the size of your average account and your clients' payment history.

3. Convert inventory to cash

I have always believed in buying large orders if I can use the inventory within six months and if the savings will be more than the interest I could earn during a similar period of time by hold-ing the money in a savings account. I know that accountants and others will disagree; however, fast turnover times look good only on paper. Fast-turnover-time accounting does not consider the high costs of being out of product and dealing with back-orders.

In times of a cash-flow crunch, you may want to sell your excess inventory to colleagues or return excess inventory to your suppliers for credit. Then begin an austerity program of careful ordering and careful use of supplies. With this new inventory pol-icy you may be able to reduce your inventory investment by as much as 50 percent.

4. Sell and lease-back your tangible property

Lease companies are usually willing to purchase your equip-ment, office furniture and vehicles at full value and lease them back to you for 24 to 60 months. Do not forget that you may have capital gains taxes to pay as well as high interest rates. This procedure is best done early in the taxable year.

Reducing expenses

by Jan Coody, MBA, Hospital Administrator at Woodland PetCare Centers

You need to challenge every cost in your business! Competition makes every price negotiable.

Meaningful cost reduction must be approached objectively with specific realistic goals. Review your financial statements from the last three to four years to identify the areas where costs have risen. Use these areas as a starting place to consider ways to reduce costs. Reducing costs needs to be an ongoing task and should receive top-of-the-mind awareness in all of your transactions. Even seemingly insignificant cost increases (or decreases!) add up to a sizable amount over time.

Staff involvement

Everyone today needs to be a cost-conscious consumer. The key to implementing effective cost reduction in your practice is to involve your personnel. Suggestions from employees are extremely effective, as these people are on the front line and know your business. They usually have many ideas for ways to save, but they need to be given incentives to make suggestions and carry out the ideas. Ask them for cost-cutting ideas, not just ideas or suggestions in general. Offer rewards for ideas that are actually used. Rewards could be a percentage of the savings, a flat dollar amount, movie tickets or dinner certificates. Make a big deal of their efforts and let them know they are appreciated.

At Woodland PetCare Centers, we present awards at our monthly staff meetings and announce them in our in-house newsletters. Announcements posted on a bulletin board can also recognize cost-cutting achievements.

Have your employee management team consider all of the ideas suggested and how to implement the ones that would work. Recognize all of the employees that participate, even if the idea is not used. Let them know you appreciate their input and tell them why the idea was not used. Ask them to keep thinking about other ways to cut costs and to keep the good ideas coming!

Office expenses

In reviewing our financial statements at Woodland PetCare Centers, some of the largest and fastest growing expenses are in the area of office expense.

Service contracts: We have saved a great deal by not using service contracts. On highly reliable equipment, in particular, they are a waste of money. The service contracts would have cost much more than the repairs. On our computer equipment we have a savings account for repairs and replacements in which we make a monthly deposit.

Auctions for office equipment and furniture: When you need office furniture and fixtures, attend your local auctions. It may mean a few late nights, but the savings can be quite sizable. By buying brand name used equipment and furniture, you will probably end up with better quality than if you purchased new. Also, companies going out of business have auctions or sales where you can even find usable supplies at a fraction of the retail cost.

Used computers: An independent computer repair person can be valuable to your office. Independents usually charge less per hour and can be very helpful with upgrading your current computers and finding parts. They can even come up with enough parts to put together a whole PC and will usually take your parts as a trade-in. There are firms that broker used equipment, and some publish catalogs of their goods. There are companies that refurbish laser cartridges. Check these out carefully, as they sometimes don't work as well or last long enough to be a real savings.

A good use for an old PC and printer is to set it up with mailing labels or checks so that you don't have to switch back and forth on your regular equipment.

Office supplies: It helps to have one employee in charge of ordering office supplies; otherwise, a lot of duplication takes place. This person can compare prices and check out the discount office supply stores and catalogs. There is usually a savings if you buy in larger quantities. Don't be tempted to buy more than is needed; but getting as much as a year's worth of cheap low-use items could be worthwhile. Ordering in standard size lots rather than splitting a box of supplies will cost less. Keeping all supplies in one location helps to see what is available and what needs to be ordered. Have all employees help gather supplies for this location. Even have them check their pockets and homes, as pens are easy to carry off.

Be sure when ordering from catalogs to take the freight cost into consideration. When you add in the freight costs, it might cost less to purchase from your office supply store.

Copying vs. printing: Figure out what it costs to photocopy a page on your copy machine. Most are 10–15 cents for paper, toner, maintenance, overhead, and labor. Taking them to your printing company can be 3–5 cents. When we need more than 15–20 copies of an item, we take it to the printer rather than use our copy machine.

Use your bulletin board to post messages rather than making copies for everyone. A board near the time clock is usually seen by everyone. Or better yet, use electronic mail on your computer.

When using your fax machine, make sure the cover sheet is plain, as it takes valuable time for one with designs to go through the machine. Another option is to use the small fax information stickers.

Subscription services: Using a magazine subscription service has been a big help to us. It is very confusing in a multi-doctor hospital to know what subscriptions we have and when they come due. The service sends a list of what we have ordered and a bill to cover all subscriptions.

We have chosen to have this sent to us once a year in December. The service we use is EBSCO Reception Room Services, Top of Oak Mountain, P.O. Box 830460, Birmingham, AL 35283.

Unnecessary forms: Once a year, have a committee review your forms. Get rid of ones that you are not using, and see which ones might be combined. To make sure forms are clear, check with clients to see what they think. Unclear forms lead to misinformation, which can cause confusion that takes time to clear up.

Personnel

Absenteeism: Unexpected absences by employees cost a great deal, both directly and indirectly. Keep records on employees' absences, and look for Monday and Friday absences. Asking the employees about this pattern at least lets them know you have noticed. Have employees call in sick to a specific supervisor rather than just whoever answers the phone. We ask those calling in sick to find a replacement before calling to say they will not be in.

Rather than have a sick-leave policy that has a "use it or lose it" clause, have a personal days policy that is similar to a vacation policy. They can use this when sick or for any other time they need off. Encourage good attendance by rewarding it.

401(k)s: The 401(k) salary-reduction plan is one of the best pension plans available at this time. It used to be that only large corporations could afford to use these plans, as administration fees were so high. The 401(k) plan we use is through Principal Financial Group, a leader in business pension plans. Nine out of 10 new pension plans that they open are 401(k)s, and many are for businesses with as few as 10 employees.

Costs are cut as employees fund their own pensions through salary reductions, and then additional matching company contributions can be made at some percentage. Even a small percentage seems to be good for employee relations. At Woodland, we contribute one percent of pay, and employees may contribute up to five percent. With that program we enrolled more than 60 percent of the qualified employees.

Other pension plans that may be of interest to small businesses are the SEP (Simplified Employee Pension) and the SARSEP, which is a streamlined 401(k).

Electronic payroll: One way to cut the expense of processing a payroll is to pay electronically. The employees' checks go directly into their bank by direct deposit. There are no checks to produce and sign. Companies that pay by direct deposit also report significantly higher employee productivity on paydays because employees don't have to kill time waiting for the checks or take time off to go to the bank.

Payroll services: Payrolls are difficult to do, especially when IRS rules on depositing payroll taxes are ever-changing and penalties are very costly. The amount paid to an outside firm may seem insignificant compared with the penalties that more than 33 percent of companies have to pay each year. It is the business of outside firms to be knowledgeable on business tax requirements and stay current of the ever-changing tax laws. They will handle correspondence with the government if there is a question and assume liability and pay any penalties that result from errors they make. We have found that companies will come down 50 percent from their original price if confronted with competitive bids.

The fewer payrolls you do a year, the bigger your savings, because administrative costs are high. By changing from a weekly payroll (or even biweekly) to a semimonthly payroll, you can save 20 to 40 percent.

Temps, interns and independent contractors: One way to have a flexible work force is to fill in with temporary help. On an hour-to-hour comparison, temps seem to cost more than permanent employees; but you need to consider the costs of finding an employee, paying benefits and taxes and all of the paperwork that adds an additional 30 percent to their wages.

By hiring a temp, it also lets you see if that person fits into your organization before considering him or her for permanent employment.

Interns or preceptors from the veterinary schools can be a low-cost way to get excellent help that benefits both parties. Pre-veterinary and veterinary students make good summer help, particularly at this busiest time of the year.

Hiring independent contractors should be considered carefully. The IRS has stiff penalties for misclassifying an employee as an independent contractor. One of the key issues is how much control you have over the contract worker and whether or not that person has anything at risk in the relationship, other than the job itself.

Be sure to check on all of the IRS rules and consider having a written agreement with all independent contractors.

Annual raises: Most businesses today can't afford annual pay increases. Let employees know this is no longer possible. Increases need to be based on merit, and the key to consider here is whether the company can afford it. Give salary reviews every 18 to 24 months rather than the once customary 12 months. (See Chapter 2: Human resources, "Creating self-directed 'dream' teams" and "Developing highly committed, self-directed teams.")

Cost-cutting technology

E-mail: Electronic mail (e-mail) is becoming more popular and is an inexpensive and efficient "paperless" way to send messages directly by computer. E-mail is cheaper than any other transmission system and even more efficient than faxing. It can also lower secretarial and administrative costs because the same person creates and sends the documents. E-mail saves time also, because it tends to be less formal than fax or hard-copy documents.

Voice mail: Voice mail can be a great benefit to a busy practice. We have been using it for over two years and keep finding more and more uses for it. Even though it provides a cost savings, it can also be irritating to some clients.

Voice mail is intended to enhance service, not to replace it. Try to keep the number of choices given to callers to a minimum. We let voice mail answer only if the receptionist is on the other line and the phone rings more than a specified number of times. It is better to have it answered by the voice mail than not at all.

One beneficial feature is that doctors and staff each have their own mailbox and can give that number out for personal calls. This has been a big help to the receptionist. The time used to answer calls can be devoted to taking care of clients. Plus, the person for whom the call is intended can retrieve messages when it is convenient, rather than being interrupted at an inconvenient time. The voice mailbox activates vibrating pagers worn by the veterinarians.

We feel it is important to begin our voice-mail message by asking callers if they have an emergency. If they do, they're told to push a number that rings a big bell, which can be heard all over the hospital and answered promptly by the first person to get to the phone.

Pet tip hotline: Another use of voice mail we have recently implemented is the pet tip hotline. We advertise this service in our yellow pages ad. Callers can listen to many different tips about caring for their pets. Besides the marketing and public relations benefit, this could help relieve technicians of having to answer so many information calls, especially in the busy summer months. Each message assists the caller in reaching a receptionist or technician directly for further information or to make an appointment. (See the *Practice Workbook*, Section 11: Marketing Protocol, for scripts to specific tips.)

Teleconferencing: Many phone systems have a teleconferencing feature. Teleconferencing is one of the most cost-effective ways to communicate. It can be a substitute for costly face-to-face meetings. One of the many uses of teleconferencing is to have sales reps brief the staff on new product uses. We have even used teleconferencing to include an employee who was recuperating at home in a team meeting.

Desktop publishing: Desktop publishing lets you design and prepare your own materials for printing, which can be a big savings. Brochures, newsletters, flyers, direct-mail pieces and any other printed items you need can be designed. There are many good programs and other sources of information available. Most area junior colleges have short, inexpensive classes on how to use these programs.

Shareware: Using shareware can be a big savings for business computer programs. Shareware is "software on the honor system." You can obtain it for free to try it out. Then if you decide to continue using it, you send a small registration fee to the software's copyright owner.

It is different from public domain software, which is available for free. Shareware is comparable to the more expensive commercial software products and is of high quality. There are programs to cover all areas of business needs. The programs are available through local computer user groups, mail-order and on-line vendors.

(See Chapter 9: Managing miscellanies, "Managing high technology," to learn more about how technology can help your practice.)

Crime costs

Embezzlement: Embezzlement is difficult to deal with, as it involves someone in a position of trust; but according to statistics, it happens frequently. You should be wary of embezzlement and let your employees know you are paying attention. Have checks and balances in place.

Try to make sure no one employee has complete authority over the money. Establish separation of financial responsibility so that the person who collects the money does not make the deposit or do the bookkeeping. The person who does the bookkeeping should not be able to sign checks. Have more than one person reconcile bank statements and review documentation. Go over the canceled checks and spot-check bank deposits. Be sure that employees who handle money are bonded.

In interviewing prospective employees, I ask them if they are willing to be bonded and let them think I am going to check this out before hiring. This helps eliminate hiring the wrong person in the first place. I have had interviewees call me back to explain about something in their past that might interfere with their being bonded. In such cases, it is best to probably keep on looking if there is any question in this area.

The Council of Better Business Bureaus lists the following warning signs to help you be aware of embezzlement:

- Accounting, inventory or other company books that are not being kept up to date by the responsible employee.

- Client invoices habitually being mailed late.

- Frequent complaints by clients that invoices are inaccurate.

- Employees who regularly turn down promotions or refuse to take time off.

- Employees who frequently ask for cash advances on paychecks.

- Employees whose standards of living are much higher than their salaries would be expected to support.

- Frequent inventory shortages.

- Slow collections, which may indicate that payments are being sidetracked on the way to the bank.

- Unusual bad-debt write-offs by bookkeeping.

***Burglaries*:** Having a good security system can save money in two ways: less theft and lower insurance rates. With some insurance companies: the better the system, the bigger the savings. Preferably, each employee should have a separate security code. That way they know that you will know when they have been in the building after hours.

***Telemarketing scams*:** Be alert to frequent calls from telemarketers. It seems the main calls we get are concerning office supplies. Some callers offer prizes and all kinds of incentives for us to order worthless supplies, which might never even arrive. A frequent scam we hear is someone informing us of an impending price increase on toner cartridges for the copy machine and then telling us we can get in an order "today" before the increase takes place.

The salespeople make it sound as if they know you and have been doing business with your organization for years. They say they are calling to confirm an order placed by someone else at your company, and in the process they get information about your business. Then they will even send invoices for goods that were never ordered and threaten collection action if those invoices are not paid.

We once had an unsuspecting receptionist order "sticky notes" at about three times the cost we normally paid at the local office supply. Not only this; but they kept sending them in monthly installments, and we had a terrible time getting them stopped because they had a recording of her agreeing to try them.

To avoid being taken in by these scams, set up a policy that no one in your office is to make any such purchases by phone. They are to always ask for further information before making purchase decisions and should not give out credit card numbers or any other information to an unknown caller. Telephone scam artists are masters at posing as the dealer or supplier calling to verify key information as to equipment make or model so they can then send bogus orders and invoices.

Energy costs

Energy-saving ideas: Cutting monthly energy costs can add to your bottom line. Many utility companies will audit your business for free or for a small fee to help you with energy conservation. Some utility companies give rebates for investing in energy-saving technology. You might consider improving the efficiency of your lighting, water heater, heating, ventilation and air-conditioning systems.

There are inexpensive devices that automatically turn lights off and on when they sense a person has entered the area. These can be installed in storage rooms, rest rooms, hallways and stairways. Their manufacturers claim their installation can cut some lighting costs by 50 percent.

Standard light bulbs can be replaced with compact fluorescent bulbs. We recently replaced our standard fluorescent bulbs with this new type of bulb. It gives off a brighter, whiter light (like being outside), and is especially good in exam rooms and areas where a lot of paperwork is done. The bulbs are expensive, but they are guaranteed to last up to seven years and save as much as 75 percent on energy costs over their lifetime. Also, there are devices that reflect fluorescent light. They are inexpensive and will boost lighting efficiency, thereby allowing you to use less energy.

Review lighting locations, too. Many fixtures are not placed where they are needed. By placing them closer to where they will be most useful, you may find you need fewer lights.

Make use of air-conditioning economizers. Your old system will work more efficiently. Newer systems may already be equipped with an economizer. Check to see if it is working properly. When it is cool and dry, the economizer tells the system to begin drawing outside air in rather than spending money cooling the warmer inside air.

Programmable thermostats can be installed at minimal cost to replace the regular ones. It is best to designate one person to be in charge of setting the thermostats and not have each employee turning them up or down according to individual desires. With zoned heating and air conditioning, it's not uncommon to find air conditioning running in one part of the hospital and heating running in another part of the hospital in the spring and fall.

Recycling: Recycling lets you cut costs in three ways:

- Less waste can mean lower disposal costs;
- Materials sold to recyclers produce cash; and
- By demonstrating that recycling is important, you encourage employees to look for other ways to conserve.

We have a place to crush and save aluminum cans in the employees' lounge. The money we get from turning them in goes to help with our Christmas party. Some firms have had considerable savings by recycling office paper, glass, magazines, junk mail and plastic.

Disposal costs: Be sure you are not overpaying your trash service. If you have used the same company for more than three years, shop around and compare prices to see if they are still in line. Fees are based on the size of the container and frequency of the trips. Do not use a container that is too big for your needs.

Check to see if it is filling up, and reduce your pickups to as few as possible per week. Luckily, our trash service called us and suggested that from their experience we could cut back from three pickups a week to two and benefit from the savings.

Telephone costs

Long-distance services: With so many long-distance companies vying for your business, it is worth reviewing your long-distance carrier at least every other year. AT&T's "Partners in Business" program offers discounts of up to 20 percent for small companies that spend between $25 and $2,000 per month.

For signing an 18-month contract, you can take another 20 percent off calls to whichever area code you call the most. MCI's "Friends of the Firm" program offers large discounts in return for the right to contact the numbers your office calls to solicit their business. Be sure to get permission from your friends first.

You also can get discounts through business affiliations. Phone companies are making strategic alliances with big banks, trade associations and other business groups under which the company or organization offers its customers or members discounted long-distance service.

There are many long-distance resellers, also called "aggregators," that buy big blocks of phone time from AT&T or other phone firms at a discount, then resell the time to smaller businesses, passing along part of the discount. We have recently affiliated with General Electric's AT&T service to receive discounted service. One advantage to using a reseller is that the giant companies are billed in six-second increments by long-distance carriers rather than the one-minute increment that is standard for smaller customers. This can add up to a 20 to 40 percent savings, depending on your phone usage.

Offers are constantly changing in this field. We regularly receive calls from the marketing departments of the various long-distance companies with various plans and offers. Pick one you like, and tell everybody else to call you back in two years.

Directory assistance: Directory assistance calls are no longer a free service. Phone companies now generate revenues of over $2 billion from those who would rather call for assistance than look up the number. Remember to check this on your phone bill and see how much you are paying per month for this service.

The cost of the average directory assistance call has crept up to about 65 cents. To reduce or eliminate this cost, make sure you receive enough free phone books. Most computers have a program for telephone numbers. You can also just make use of the old standby, Rolodex® card file. Automatic dial features on your phone system will also minimize the use of directory assistance.

Phone bills: Phone companies can make mistakes, so audit your phone bill regularly. Check out any questionable numbers. Do not forget to include your cellular phone bill in your audit. Errors in this bill are even more common. We had an instance where a hang-up was not recognized and $370.00 was charged to the bill.

Do a cost accounting of phone calls. Some phone companies will provide you with this service, or there are companies that specialize in this area. This cost-accounting plan groups monthly phone activities so you can see what is happening. It lets you see where the calls are going, how long they are lasting, who is making them and when. This lets you spot bad calling habits that are costing you money and helps you spot phone abuse, too.

Many companies are opting to receive an electronic version of their phone bill. By adding it to billing management software, you can quickly analyze the bill.

The phone company (for a fee) will do a busy-signal study for you. This lets you see if you are missing calls and need to add an additional line.

Pagers versus cellular phones: Compared with personal and car cellular phones, the pager seems mundane. But if it will fit your needs, for a much lower cost it may be the best choice. Pager prices depend on the type you choose. Tone-only pagers are cheapest. They alert you to a message but don't tell you what it is. Numeric pagers, the most popular, have a tiny screen that displays up to 20 digits, usually the phone number of where you can return the call. Alphanumeric pagers have a larger screen and let you receive a full message without having to return the call.

Fax: Most fax machines can be programmed to send faxes at certain hours. By sending long-distance faxes at night, you benefit from the lower rates. A savings of 20 to 40 percent can be seen on long-distance charges.

Accounting and legal costs

Detailed billing: Invoices for accounting and legal services are very brief, such as "prepare contract correspondence, $500."

By demanding detailed billing, you have a better chance of monitoring and lowering costs. Ask for bills that state what work was done, who performed the work, how long it took and what the hourly rate was. This way you can more easily spot errors, see where the money is going and look for areas where you might save. Challenge any questionable costs. Monitor the bill and let the accountant or lawyer know you are scrutinizing costs. This can spur them to watch more closely what they do or even lower their costs. By taking a closer look at the invoices, you may think twice before making lengthy telephone conversations or visiting with your accountant. Phone calls usually tend to be less expensive than personal visits. Meetings tend to ramble on, especially if several people are involved.

If others need to be involved, consider the teleconferencing feature of the phone. Have questions ready ahead of time, and have several people take notes so there is less chance of forgetting or misinterpreting something.

Independent firms audit legal and accounting bills for a fee, if you feel such a service is justified. They look for errors, waste and inefficiencies.

Fees: Most accountants' and lawyers' fees are negotiable. Try to negotiate flat rates for routine work. If you pay a retainer, look for a price break over the non-retainer rate. Use a retention letter or litigation engagement contract that lists the work to be done, what you expect and what you will and will not pay. Ask accountants to be sure and utilize their trained assistants as much as possible.

Summary

Regardless of the size of your practice or your financial status, one of the best ways to make money is to save it. How well you manage your spending affects profits more than how much you bring in. To maximize profits, consider all possible ways to cut overhead and increase productivity. Manage "leaner;" negotiate harder. In order to survive, businesses of all sizes are downsizing and doing what it takes to become more effective and competitive.

Source:

Kehrer, D. M. *Save Your Business A Bundle*. New York: Simon & Schuster, 1994.

Controlling insurance costs

by Ross D. Clark, DVM

My experience tells me that veterinarians can save themselves hundreds of dollars, year after year, by investing just a little of their limited management time in the area of insurance. A one-time decision there can save you thousands of premium dollars over the years. So let's dig out those insurance policies (from a fireproof safe, I hope) and review them one by one.

Life insurance

Insurance companies say the higher our income and the more our worth, the more life-insurance protection we need to provide to ensure our families can continue to live in the style to which they have become accustomed. Life insurance companies and their agents have repeated this rhetoric for so long that the amount of life insurance proposed is often not a sound business judgment but an amount based upon your income, emotion and insurance company charts. Competent financial planners present the argument that a wealthy person needs less life insurance than a less affluent and usually younger person. What insurance agents are really saying is that veterinarians can usually afford to pay the higher premiums.

Let us for the moment continue to assume that the more prosperous person wants to leave more to his family. We still are not talking about insurance needs but capital needs. A person with a net worth of $600,000 and a $40,000 annual income needs less life insurance than a person with a net worth of $100,000 and a $60,000 income.

Of course, life insurance needs also depend on the number of children you have, how old they are, how old you are and your spouse's prospects for gainful employment and/or re-marriage once you're gone. Don't forget Social Security benefits that accrue to families at the death of a spouse.

Harvey Sarner, a well-known tax and estate planner, often says, "I don't understand doctors having such high life insurance values unless they want their wives to have happy second husbands." Married veterinarians, male or female, need to consult with their spouses soon and discuss whether they need these premium dollars more now or later. If you are single, of course your insurance needs are less; however, don't forget that you could later become uninsurable.

Life insurance policies have been a source of many "surprises" recently, especially cash-value policies that have been stung by declines in interest rates. Cash-value policies combine insurance with a tax-deferred savings feature. With some policies, some of the earnings are used to pay premiums or build a nest egg for retirement.

People who bought certain policies usually received an estimate of how much their policy could be worth over time, through the use of policy "illustrations" or "projections." But when the policies were sold, interest rates were higher. Now, because rates are much lower, those projections may be grossly overstated.

Veterinarians may find themselves paying premiums for longer than they anticipated and maybe even paying higher premiums, or they may find out that their retirement fund is not as large as they thought it would be. Ask your agent for an "insurance ledger," showing how your policy is doing currently; and compare that with where it should be, based on the projection made when the policy was purchased. If there's a gap, you could be in for some surprises. If the projections are about the same, you can sleep soundly at night.

As for other details of a life insurance policy, it's important to know who the owner is. The owner is the one who can make changes in the policy. When one spouse is the owner of the policy and the other spouse is the beneficiary (the one who receives the death benefits). In the case of divorce the owner spouse can change the beneficiary. For the protection of the beneficiary, the beneficiary and the owner should be the same.

Other life insurance provisions that could stand a closer look:

- *Waiver of premium* allows you to stop paying premiums and still be covered if you're disabled. It might be okay if you don't have a disability policy; but otherwise, don't get it because of the extra cost.

- *Accidental death riders* pay twice the death benefit if you die in an accident. If you need twice as much insurance, get that much coverage in the first place and don't pay extra for accidental death.

- *Claims payments* can differ by company. Some companies pay off in two weeks to a month, but most companies have up to a year to pay a claim.

You should always buy either term or universal life insurance because the premiums are significantly lower. Independent financial planners agree that whole life insurance policies are a poor place to put your savings and investments. If you currently have a whole life policy, it's a good idea to purchase a paid-up policy and convert to decreasing term or a universal life policy that combines a term insurance plan plus an investment portion currently yielding eight to 10 percent nontaxable annual return.

Auto insurance

Consider dropping collision coverage if your car isn't financed (or if the lender will agree). Save the premium instead. *Caution*: odds are always in the owner's favor to self-insure. How do you think insurance companies build those big buildings and insurance agents often make more than we do? However, risk remains. You should only self-insure if you can handle the repair cost of a major collision.

If you are not comfortable with self-insurance, the next best option would be to select a policy with a high deductible.

Real and personal property

Most property insurance contracts require the insured to purchase a policy which covers 80 percent or more of the actual value of the property. This is called co-insurance and is difficult to avoid. Most policies will pay the full value of the property destroyed only if the insured value is below 80 percent or more of the replacement value of the real estate. If coverage is below 80 percent, the maximum payment is limited to replacement value minus a depreciation charge (usually quite large).

You can still safely cut costs by building fire walls and installing fire, smoke and burglar alarms. If you are building or remodeling, be sure to use steel beams, rock, brick and concrete blocks when possible.

The use of these materials can cut insurance costs by as much as 50 percent. And, by the way, you, your family, your employees and your customers' pets will actually be much safer.

Be sure that your property and equipment insurance policy reads "replacement cost" rather than "cash value." In the event of a fire, it may be difficult to prove actual value and you will be forced to settle for a depreciated value. Consider having income protection insurance. When we experienced our fire at Woodland PetCare Centers in 1989, this type of insurance paid us $59,000 for lost net income during the nine months following the fire. They compared our actual net income to what we could have projected from historic performance.

Home insurance

The first step in gaining a better understanding of a home-owner's policy is to take note of how broad the coverage is. A "named perils policy" insures only for losses linked to a peril specifically listed in the policy. A better option would be an "all risk policy," which covers all perils unless specifically excluded. Some policies might be "all risk" on the dwelling but "named perils" on the contents.

The second area to look at is "loss settlement provisions." That section will tell you whether your losses will be covered for "actual cash value" or "replacement cost." With actual cash value, the value of your property is calculated at a depreciated value, taking into account the age of the property. If you have a seven-year-old dining room set with a 10-year life, you'll get 30 cents on the dollar.

Replacement-cost coverage does not depreciate the property for age, and the insurance company typically will pay the cost of replacing the old property with new property (subject to any restrictions). Insurance agents generally advise replacement-cost coverage, which is only $5 to $10 a year more than actual cash value.

Other potential pitfalls:

- *Check the "endorsements" section or "special limits of liabilities"* because even if you have replacement-cost coverage, some contents—such as paintings, antiques or other collectibles—might not be eligible. Specifically, a riding mower might be covered but not a child's dirt bike.

- *The method of payment can vary.* With some companies you might get paid up front; but with other companies, you might need to replace your property first, then get reimbursed. Being reimbursed is less desirable than being paid up front.

- *You might incur some out-of-pocket expenses* under a "co-insurance penalty," which kicks in with a partial loss if you don't insure a dwelling for at least 80 percent of its reconstruction value. With a total loss, you would receive

up to the policy limits. Make sure you insure for reconstruction value, not simply market value. To be safe, ask
your agent for a "replacement cost estimator."

Accident, health and disability insurance

In today's hi-tech, bypass, transplant, MRI and linear accelera-
tor society, medical insurance is the most complex, most
expensive and most important type of insurance. The complexi-
ties of these insurance policies and the rapid changes within our
society dictate that you buy your medical insurance from a large,
stable company you can trust; then leave it there.

Many health insurance programs operated by state veterinary
medical associations have folded, sometimes leaving their policy-
holders looking for alternative insurance. Some of these members
will be restricted to buying policies that exclude coverage of an
expensive and chronic health situation, such as a cardiovascular
problem or a chronic orthopedic problem. AVMA's area ratings
will give you the strength of a national organization with strong
reserves at a premium rate commensurate with health-care costs
in your area.

The best way to save money is to elect for one of the high-
deductible options. Deductibles up to $50,000 (yes, $50,000) are
available unless you are already a heavy user of insurance or
expect to be.

Health insurance plans are especially complicated and
involved; but at the very least, review the following areas:

- *Understand the "preexisting condition" clause.* Most policies will not pay for an illness or an injury for which you
  have been treated in the past 12 months. Some policies,
  PPOs and groups are more liberal, with clauses allowing a
  three- or six-month preexisting condition or even a current condition (including pregnancy). Check around.

- *Check to see if there is a waiting period for certain
  expenses*, such as with a pregnancy. For example, a policy

may cover expenses related to a pregnancy, but not if it occurs within the first six months of coverage.

- *Determine your maximum out-of-pocket expenses* for a given year.

- *Find out the policy's lifetime maximum,* such as $1 million, $2 million or unlimited.

- *Don't buy any health policy or subscribe to any group without shopping around.* Lately, the health insurance business has been changing daily.

Considerable savings can be made on disability insurance by having disability payments start as long as possible after the injury. By taking a disability policy with a 90-day waiting period, you save as much as 20 percent over a similar plan with a 30-day waiting period.

Employee medical benefits

Extend the waiting period for new employees to be eligible for medical benefits from 30 to 90 days, especially in high turnover jobs. Research shows that many people take a job specifically for the medical benefits, especially part-time help. With a longer waiting period, you'll eliminate or reduce such applicants.

Workman's compensation

If you are a sole proprietor, partner or stockholder and have adequate life, health and disability insurance, you have the option not to insure yourself under Workman's Compensation in most states.

Many owner veterinarians are unnecessarily "double-insured" in this area; and by discounting your coverage, you will be able to realize considerable savings. People with clerical jobs are covered at a lower rate than those working with animals. Be sure that a fair portion of your assistants are listed as clerical help on your policy. This will lower your rates.

Summary

There are at least 30 different kinds of insurance that a veterinarian might want to consider. This report discusses only the types of insurance most likely to result in savings. When considering the other types, try to self-insure a high portion of each. Cover yourself for the big expense and save for the small expenses.

I know of one large veterinary hospital owner who self-insured his staff for all health and accident coverage up to $50,000 per year. The first year they experienced the largest claim in their history ($30,000). At the end of two years, he still had a savings by adopting the self-insurance plan.

Make an appointment with a broker you can trust, and spend two or three hours of quality time attempting to cut your premiums by using the methods mentioned in this chapter and by eliminating as many overlaps in your insurance programs as possible.

Insurance brokers and agents can be a big help. Most of them are there to give you their honest evaluation of what is best for you; however, we must remember that they are constantly exposed to the positive side of the insurance issue and tend to encourage you to over-insure. It's up to you to periodically review your insurance program and compare coverage and premiums. If your current agent or broker gives you good service and pays your claims, and if the competitive premiums are not more than 10 percent less overall, you should stay with your current company.

Notes

Chapter 4:
Marketing, Advertising and Public Relations

Contemporary marketing

by Ross D. Clark, DVM

Marketing will be the driving force of the near future of veterinary medicine.

Practice success in the near future will only come to those of us who become formidable marketers. Veterinarians are running out of leverage. Profitable vaccines, ovariohysterectomies, castrations and declaws have been reduced to a commodity. We must learn how to differentiate our services from these average or standard veterinary services. It's a common misconception worldwide that having the best product or service practically guarantees success. In reality, some of the best products ever made have failed in the marketplace because of flawed or non-existent marketing programs. Certainly some of the best services ever offered have gone unnoticed by the general public simply because they weren't marketed properly.

If you are in any profession or service business today you are also in the marketing business. Marketing separates the good product from other good products. Marketing separates the good service from other good services. Master marketer Jay Abraham recently made the following observation: "Businesses not marketing driven, no matter how good their products or services and no matter how well managed, either go broke or struggle to survive. On the other hand, most every business that is marketing driven tends to be successful regardless of otherwise mediocre management. Of course the biggest successes came from companies that have good products and/or services, are well managed and are market driven."

Marketing must educate our potential customers to appreciate our inherent value by giving customers the "inside story" of our business so it comes to life and has more credibility in their mind. When we adequately inform someone before asking them to buy, it adds dimension to the perceived value of our product or service.

In 1919, Schlitz Beer was the first beer company to explain how their beer was made. They told about the 12 pounds of barley in every six-pack and how each batch was tasted and re-tasted seven different times before being shipped. Although all beer was made that way, Schlitz pre-empted all other competition and sales soared.

Ask other businesses in your town to help you advertise your practice. Example: Ask your local travel agent to place a "$10 off your first boarding visit" coupon in with airline and cruise tickets. The travel agency gets the credit for helping their clients with "dollars-off" coupons and you get economical advertising even when clients don't use the coupons right away. And we shouldn't forego marketing opportunities at our own place of business.

Reception room marketing

- We can differentiate our clinics and our services by emphasizing our experience. Tell about the length of employee service. Appeal to the cautious side of clients by asking them indirectly not to risk changing to those less experienced.

- We could elaborate on how carefully we select and train our staff.

- We need to feature pictures of our staff with their pets in the reception area.

- We need pictures of our clients' champion dogs and grand champion cats in the reception area "wall of fame."

- We should post photographs of our staff veterinarians and their pets. And we must include their resume and personal information so that clients can know more about us and bond with our practice and our staff, because of shared experiences: that fact that we too own a greyhound or a boxer, or a Siamese or Persian cat; or that we also attended OSU, KSU, or Notre Dame; or the same local high school; or because we have hobbies in common, etc.

- We should educate our clients. Our practice has purchased several copies of Dr. Rooks Slocum's composite X-ray film comparing radiographs of hip dysplasia to a normal canine pelvis, for instance; and we display these in the exam rooms and in our reception area. Dr. Slocum created this special radiograph depicting normal hips, dysplastic hips and several ways to surgically correct dysplastic hips all on a 14 x 17 film. This special radiographic presentation can be obtained from Slocum Enterprises, Inc., 621 River Ave., Eugene, OR 97404; phone: 1-800-346-5489.

- We should entertain our clients. AVLS PetCom in Lincoln, Nebraska, has developed a reception room photo CD program (to run on a standard television), which will provide clients with a continuous visual tour of your hospital and highlight the services that you offer. We could also include photos of our veterinarians, their pets and their biography on the AVLS system. Clients hate waiting time more than fees. This program helps keep them entertained and informed at the same time. Similarly, if a client waits more than eight minutes, someone should talk to him. This will give you another eight minutes before the client becomes impatient.

- We should offer our clients more, instead of cutting our prices. Write them, call them, send information—maintain "top of the mind" awareness. Be sure that our names, addresses and telephone numbers are on everything that leaves our clinics and hospitals including our delivery van. A properly identified van on the street with our logo on its side can be as effective as an outdoor billboard to maintain "top of the mind" awareness.

- We can be on time. The organization and efficiency of the practice is questionable when a veterinarian isn't on time for a scheduled appointment. Clients are concerned about their problems, not the problems of a veterinarian who can't stay organized and on time. Clients feel that you are too busy and feel that you just don't need their business. Some tardiness is excusable, but there are very few good reasons to be late.

Focus group study

New City Marketing sent a comprehensive questionnaire to 600 of Woodland PetCare Centers' clients, called 200 of those clients and then held a focus group study with 15 of them. The resulting study found the following desires prevalent among our clients:

- convenience (open seven days a week);

- quality care;

- 24-hour care;

- veterinarians and staff members who know unique characteristics of all their pets;

- veterinarians who listen;

- veterinarians who make rounds for difficult cases; and

- clinics that reward client loyalty with some kind of a frequent buyer program.

Wayne Blackman, president of New City Marketing, says that we must never assume that even our very best clients know about all of the services we have to offer. We must market to our existing clients for a bigger piece of the client. I hold no stock in the AVLS systems, but I believe that their program fits very well into Wayne Blackman's recommendation.

What it takes

The average business spends six times as much to acquire a new client as it takes to keep a current client. Veterinary medicine is somewhat intangible. We must make it more tangible by:

- building a quality facility;

- developing quality personnel;

- wearing quality uniforms; and

- sending out only quality written materials.

The role of nutrition in marketing

by Ross D. Clark, DVM

As competition for the pet-care dollar continues to increase, we must take another look at the role of pet nutrition in marketing to our existing clients. Don Peppers and Martha Rogers, Ph.D., in their book, *The One to One Future ... Building Relationships, One Customer at a Time* (New York: Doubleday, 1993), point out that a bigger piece of the market pie has become more and more difficult to achieve. However, a larger share of the individual customer may be available to help us maintain profitability and growth.

We, as veterinarians, are the best qualified to give nutritional advice to our clients. I believe that good nutrition is the medication of the next millennium. Dr. Jacob Mosier, a recognized authority in the field of canine and feline gerontology, reports that cats and dogs would commonly live to be 24 years old if they had optimum nutrition and dental care from day one. There is opportunity for veterinarians to save your good clients worry and time regarding what diet to feed their pets.

New prescription diets

Veterinary prescribed diets that provide treatment as well as prevention are becoming available for more and more medical problems. It's clear to me that a client who purchases a lifetime of prescribed diets will provide substantial income to your practice not only from the direct sales of foods, but secondary sales of other health care products. We also develop tertiary revenue from the increased awareness of our clinic's or hospital's services, created by the clients increased visits. Wayne Blackman of New City Marketing in Tulsa says that "we must never assume that even our very best clients know everything about all of the services we have available."

Some veterinarians are hesitant about "selling" wellness diets. If the term "selling" bothers you, substitute the word "offering." By not offering wellness diets you may actually inconvenience your clients—they may prefer "one-stop shopping"—while depriving your patients of optimum health through proper nutrition. Additionally, by distributing trial-size food samples and "money-back" rebate certificates, you may get the credit for saving your clients money while food manufacturers foot the bill.

I recommend selling staff members prescribed diet foods at cost. When staff members feed their pets the food they become ambassadors for the product. Be sure to give your staff plenty of training and to reward them for taking and passing nutrition courses sponsored by manufacturers.

Clients want a professional to recommend what's best for their treasured companion. People feel good about taking that companion to the best doctor in town and providing him or her with the best foods available.

Veterinary prescribed diets are the only pet food products that do not put veterinary practices in direct competition with pet stores and "super stores." Do not attempt to compete on price. Compete on convenience and service. Touting proper nutrition has more client appeal than being a "pill pusher," "vitamin salesman" or "injection king."

Clients want a professional to recommend what's best for their treasured companion. People feel good about taking that companion to the best doctor in town and providing him or her with the best foods available.

Veterinarians currently only capture three to seven percent of the potential pet food market from their client base, which usually represents about three to eight percent of their total gross. Some veterinarians have boosted their prescribed diets sales to 15 percent of their total gross, or more. If your practice is grossing three percent from prescribed diet sales, you have the potential of at least 10 percent growth in your gross by actively offering quality nutrition for your client's pets. In other words, a practice grossing $500,000 could increase the gross by $50,000 and the bottom line by $15,000 by increasing prescribed food sales. Your gross and net will also be enhanced by the increased visits to your practice and by increased awareness of your practice and the services you offer.

The more comprehensive the assortment of products and services a business supplies, the less likely you'll be seen as a commodity. No other health-related product or service will bring clients into your hospital or clinic as often as veterinary prescribed diets. Superstores have developed their high volume of business because customers return again and again for pet food. Superstores have based their success on a premise that veterinarians discarded over and over as a waste of time, space and resources. We can still recover and then recapture market and client share by making veterinary prescribed diets an integral part of our canine and feline wellness programs.

Marketing ideas collage

by Ross D. Clark, DVM, and Ron Whitford, DVM, mixed animal practitioner and owner of three clinics in Clarksville, Tenn.

Marketing does not just sell products and services. It coordinates all things that shape the public's image of your clinic.

The marketing of veterinary services can be divided into external and internal areas of application. Internal marketing targets existing clients. It includes client communications, hospital appearance, reminders, diversification of profit centers, etc. External marketing programs are directed outside the practice, targeting non-clients and nonusers of veterinary medical services. Our profession should concentrate most of its marketing efforts on internal marketing techniques catering to clients already using our services. It is always easier to sell to those that already buy.

We do not, as individual practitioners, generate sufficient revenue to buy media advertising that will have a significant impact on the public at large. We need to perfect our services to current clients since there still are very few veterinary practices that can boast of having the majority of patients up-to-date on all the preventive health care recommendations suggested. We don't need to service more clients superficially. We need to provide more complete service to existing clients.

Be first! Marketing consultants Al Reis and Jack Trout point out that it's better to be first than it is to be better. As an example, who was the second person to fly the Atlantic ocean solo?

We all know that Lindbergh was first. Bert Hinkler was second—he flew faster and used less fuel, but we don't remember his name. If you want to know which college is first, just substitute "leading" for first, and you have your answer—Harvard. In the same manner, *Time* leads *Newsweek; People* magazine leads *US* magazine; *Playboy* leads *Penthouse*; the ever-popular *TV Guide* still remains unchallenged; and Chrysler still leads in mini-vans.

Distribute creative business cards:

- Use a professionally designed logo.

- Use color discretely to give your card more impact.

- Use the back of the card. It costs almost nothing and it is otherwise wasted space. You can use the back of your card as a mini-brochure. You could have a map showing how to find your clinic or hospital.

- Use a fold-over card to do the same things as the back of your card and more.

- Consider having your card also serve as a Rolodex® card.

- Consider investing in a software program that will allow you to get creative and make your own cards on your computer.

Know your own worth. We must first convince ourselves of our worth and the value of the services we provide. After we have convinced ourselves of our worth, we must convince the staff— and then the clients.

The best salesperson in veterinary medicine is the veterinarian who knows and appreciates the value of the services he or she is capable of providing. To be successful, you must provide and market services and products on which you, yourself, are sold. With the right attitude and philosophy, clients will want your services without a "hard sell." Give the client enough information to make an educated decision.

Use direct mail. Again, Reis and Trout say, "It's better to be first in the mind than it is to be first in the marketplace." Try to maintain top-of-the-mind awareness. Keep your name out there in the public eye.

One low-priced way to keep clients reminded of your name and location is to send them newsletters. They tell your clients that, "You are a member of our club, no matter how the rest of your social life is going." Newsletters can be a good source of information. By sending newsletters you will gain increased respect and loyalty from your existing client base. Newsletters are effective because they can be targeted—first to current clients, second to the breed of pet they own.

Another effective direct-mail technique is to send pieces that combine general information about staff and other activities in your clinic with a very targeted section about the clients' particular breed of cat or dog.

Project an image. Marketing is not a battle of products and services. It's a battle of perceptions! Our style of marketing program at the Woodland PetCare Centers includes researching what our market wants and then creating the impression that *that* is exactly what we offer.

We realized, for example, that our target market placed a high value on the availability of our services, so our central clinic in Tulsa is open 7 a.m. to 7 p.m. Monday through Friday, 8 a.m. to 5 p.m. on Saturdays, and 1 p.m. to 5 p.m. on Sundays and holidays. Our street sign reader board can therefore honestly announce that we are "Open 7 days a week, 365 days a year!" But a focus group study conducted for our practice by New City Marketing revealed that 12 out of 15 of our clients think we are open 24 hours a day, 365 days a year!

Always remember: The public's perception of Johnson & Johnson after the Tylenol incident was favorable—even though people died because of the tampering. Yet, the public perception of Three Mile Island was negative even though no one died.

Use an exterior sign to bring in clients. Clients decide to use a particular veterinary hospital by first becoming aware of the facility through exterior signage. They then evaluate the practice as to its ability to meet their needs, and then evaluate this ability against their expectations through a trial use of its services. If their expectations are met and exceeded, they then most often become enthusiastic marketers of the hospital. We win new clients by determining their unmet needs. Ask your current clients how you can do better. Most innovations are small incremental improvements, not "block-buster" breakthroughs.

Be happy and enthusiastic! Effective marketing of veterinary services and products requires imagination. It must change from year to year and should be fun as well as rewarding. People buy when and where it makes them feel good.

There is an art to selling services. It does not require expensive advertising, but rather simply providing clients with enough motivation and information to convince them to do what is best for their pets. Remember that 68 percent of all clients who leave a practice do so because of a "perceived" poor attitude of one or more staff members and not because of price or hard sell.

Seriously consider adding a second veterinarian to your practice, if you haven't already done so. Most solo practices can easily support another practitioner by increasing the time allotted to each case, extending hours (thus providing services at a time convenient to clients), remaining open during "lunch hours," handling more emergencies, etc.

Adding a second practitioner should also make it possible for you to devote more time to the management of your practice. Schedule time to think. Quiet time is very important. In today's competitive environment, the owner of a practice probably should spend at least 25 percent of the time in management and marketing decision making.

Emphasize services that you like to perform. This will almost ensure success. It might be internal medicine, dentistry, surgery, dermatology or endoscopy. This can aid your practice in the establishment of one or more niches for client service, specialties that lie beyond the routine exam.

The major emphasis in private practice has changed from "trauma medicine" to clinical practice from emergency medicine to internal medicine. Public leash laws, human emphasis on pre-

The major emphasis in private practice has changed from "trauma medicine" to clinical practice from emergency medicine to internal medicine. Public leash laws, human emphasis on preventive medicine and longer lifespans for pets contribute to these changes. Understand that you can market to a much larger number of clients and receive a higher fee for your services if you position yourself as a "consultant" rather than a "vendor."

Today's clients want a veterinarian who can serve as an information source that they can understand. They want a veterinarian that enjoys routine exams and interacting with pets and themselves. They want a veterinarian who is enthusiastic about healthy, well-behaved pets. Even in today's world, there still is a shortage of quality-oriented, people-oriented, caring veterinarians.

Equip yourself to do things the client cannot do. Don't depend on such things as vaccinations, which can be purchased elsewhere. Price "shopped services" competitively. You must first get the client in the door before you can market yourself, your hospital and your services.

> *Look for services you can provide more effectively, efficiently and cost-effectively for the client. Any service or convenience you can offer clients that is better for the client is a true niche for a stronger practice in the future*

Look for services you can provide more effectively, efficiently and cost-effectively for the client. Any service or convenience you can offer clients that is better for the client is a true niche for a stronger practice in the future. If a service has a purpose, offer it! Diversification of the practice by creating additional profit cen-

have to the client, the more opportunities you have for additional marketing.

Communicate with clients. We don't have to impress them. Our advice is always accepted more readily when it is offered honestly and in the "first person."

Ethical marketing raises your community profile and provides potential clients with the information they need to make educated decisions. It seeks to gain more referrals from enthusiastic clients sold on your practice. The person who stands on honesty has a good point of view. Nothing ruins the truth like stretching it. Being honest is the best practice builder.

Today, the general public perceives the veterinarian as a health care provider who serves the needs of the family pet. Our major source of income will continue to be professional veterinary knowledge and services, not products. We can only serve in that capacity if we are accurately perceived as honest practitioners.

Understand today's client. Numerous social changes over the last 25 years have had a major impact on our profession. Families are smaller and rely upon multiple wage earners. There are more senior citizens. These changes have affected the way owners value and care for their pets.

The pet-owning public is made of three distinct groups: bargain hunters who buy at the lowest price, value-benefit consumers who factor value and benefit of the services into their buying decisions and consumers who demand quality regardless of price. The middle (value-oriented) group makes up about 70 percent of the total clientele, with each of the other groups representing about 15 percent of the clientele. Purchases today are based on desire and perceived value, not need and price. We must always give more in perceived value than we take in cash value.

Today's demanding client wants to be pampered, appreciated and catered to. Practices that not only meet these needs and expectations but exceed them will thrive in the future. Clients want *value*. There are no price lists in this type of marketing. The value you provide determines the price. There are several types of "value:"

- less costly in the long term ("life cycle");
- more service for the same price ("increased productivity") and
- increased pride ("good feelings").

Young, growing families make up 50 percent of the families in the United States, and half of these households own pets. Only 12 percent of older people and singles own pets; only 18 percent of families with grown children own pets; "traditional" pets simply don't fit their life-styles.

Generally speaking, different sorts of clients have different sorts of expectations. Female clients, as a rule:

- have higher expectations of quality,
- are concerned about accuracy,
- want convenient hours and
- expect competent personnel.

Middle-aged clients, similarly:

- want easy access,
- look for reliability and
- expect competence.

And older clients:

- want courtesy,
- expect security,
- want to be recognized by name,
- expect competence,

- look for confidentiality and

- sometimes want sympathy as well.

Demographic data like this can give you great insight into the most probable groups of clients to "target" in your area. Don't spend your marketing efforts and budget on the wrong target group.

Summary

Consumer standards have risen significantly, providing grim prospects for veterinary practices that don't meet the expectations of today's potential clients. We must commit to excellence. Quality has become a prerequisite for marketing success. The "rubber meets the road" when clients come to your hospital demanding cutting-edge technology. Your hospital's technological prowess then becomes an issue of competition and fiscal survival. Clients will desire more service as pet value increases.

We must market total health care. Annual physical examinations create a niche unique to the veterinary professional. We are the ones trained to perform a thorough examination. It is estimated that a pet has at least two and half problems for every problem for which it is presented.

Most practices can stay busy simply by performing thorough examinations and then making recommendations based on those findings. We must learn to focus on health, not disease. Recent evidence suggests that the American public is more concerned with preventive care than are many veterinarians.

Ten-step exam room protocol to bond clients to your practice

by Ross D. Clark, DVM

The majority of income generated in a veterinary facility starts in an examination room. This makes the examination room the most important 100 square feet in your practice. To improve your exam room sales and delivery technique, take a closer look at the examination rooms and the activity that goes on there. The time spent and the cost of upgrading are minimal when compared with the results that can be achieved. Go into one of your examination rooms and stand on the clients' side of the examination table for 20 minutes.

- What impression does this room give about the quality of medicine practiced in your clinic?

- Is it clean and in good condition?

- Is it comfortable ?

- Does it seem to be medical? Do you see stethoscopes, ophthalmoscopes, otoscopes, electronic thermometers and other medical accouterments there?

I first talked about an exam room protocol to bond clients to your practice at the Third *Veterinary Economics* Practice Management Seminar in Chicago in November 1980. That portion of my presentation remains one of the most popular segments of my seminars. Several veterinarians I know have posted these 10 steps outside each exam room door. To make a client's visit to your hospital an absolutely profound experience is challenging. Communicating is difficult, as we all know, but it can be fun as well as supremely rewarding to you and to your cash flow to get these 10 steps incorporated into every client visit to your clinic.

1. Present yourself as a medical professional.

a) Wear a white smock. Studies show that a white lab coat or smock rates 17 percent higher with clients.

b) Have a stethoscope around your neck or in your coat pocket.

c) Wear a large name badge.

d) Wash and dry your hands in the exam room.

e) Keep a charged otoscope and opthalmoscope in each exam room.

As soon as you step into the exam room, introduce yourself and shake hands with the client or clients. Come out from behind the exam table to greet them. Maintain full frontal body posture toward the client—face and body. Make eye contact as you tell them your name (write the color of their eyes on the record to confirm to yourself and others that you have in fact looked them in the eye).

"Get out of your box!" When you stand in one spot, your voice and actions tend to become robotic. Use your name and your client's name at least three times during the office call and examination. This creates a friendly yet professional atmosphere in the exam room while "Fido's" problems are addressed.

Have the animals chart in your hand so the client is aware that you know why they are here, as well as any special concerns that may have brought them in to see you. After you see a client for a number of visits, ask them to please use your first name. People love to do business with a friend.

2. Touch and talk to the client and the pet.

The conversation and hand contact between you and the clients can frequently allay the fears of the animal. Remember that most of the pets you see are cherished companions and their acceptance of you is very important to their owners. It is up to you and your technicians to instill confidence in the animal and its owners. Pet owners want you to like and care about their pets.

They must feel that their well-being is your hospital's most important function. As you discuss the pet's medical symptoms and signs with the client, pet the animal and talk to it as well.

When I ask clients why they have switched veterinarians they often tell me it was because they felt their past veterinarians did not like Dobermans or cats or their dog in particular. When I ask how they knew that, they commonly reply that they were disappointed in how little their previous veterinarian touched and talked to their pet. If the pet is in serious condition, and the time seems appropriate, touch the top of your clients hand when you tell them the news.

3. Do something medical.

Now is the time to reinforce their opinion of you as a professional. Begin to address the animal medically. You may listen to the heart and respiration, eyeball a laceration or skin problem or have the technician do a collection for a fecal float. While you are doing any kind of examining, be sure to continue to talk in a quiet tone that not only soothes the animal but keeps the client apprised of what you are doing.

Every exam room in America should have the proper accouterments clients expect in a medical facility—including a rechargeable ophthalmoscope and otoscope. These instruments should be used to check each patient during each office visit, and the findings reported to the client. Remember clients love to hear that their pets are normal and healthy. They want to hear that their dog has a strong heart, eyes free of cataracts or any retinal problems and ears that are clean and free of infection. If you're going to do a procedure that looks hurtful or one that is hurtful, forewarn the client. If an animal seems highly fractious, ask the owner's permission to remove the animal to a treatment room where it can't hide behind its owners. It usually presents a more professional image to the client.

Removing a pet from the owner can be a very delicate matter; be sure that they approve. I've witnessed a few disasters where clients, technicians and veterinarians have all been soiled with blood, feces and urine trying to trim a Chihuahua's toenails in the exam room. I'm sure that scenes like this do not help our professional image. Use this opportunity while you're out of the room to show the client a videotape on nutrition, parasites or behavior.

4. Be an active listener.

During these initial few minutes in the exam room you should be able, by watching and listening carefully, to decide what kind of client you are dealing with and to which of their senses you will need to appeal. Some of this appealing to the client for permission or agreement will depend on the type of procedure you are recommending as well as the type of client with which you are dealing. If your client has never stopped talking, he is probably an auditory person. To this person you would say, "How does that sound to you?" When you answer this client say, "That sounds good to me." Another client might be one who watches carefully everything you do; one who wants to see the treatment. If you listen to this client you will hear lots of "I see," or "I have seen" or "Do you see?" To this visual client you present your prescribed treatment with, "Can you see — ?" And you answer these clients with "I see exactly what you mean."

Yet another client may be kinesthetic, one who says little but "feels" things. If you listen to this client you will hear: "I didn't feel like he needed that" or "I felt differently." When discussing treatment or decisions with this person you nod and say, "I can understand exactly how you feel." Be a good listener, people love doing business with professionals that listen. Clients also love doing business with professionals who see, hear and feel things the way they do.

5. Say something.

As already noted, your voice can soothe both the patient and the client. A vaccine given in silence is not going to satisfy a client. He wants his money's worth for the time he spends with you. Many clients feel that you charge too much and expect good advice as well as treatment. The most important part of the vaccination process is the physical examination. It is up to the veterinarian to explain each observation to the clients. That advice serves you both well. I must re-emphasize that you should report normal findings as well as abnormal findings. People want to hear that they are doing a good job of caring for their pet.

6. Show and tell.

Now is the time to show the client something pertaining to the future good health of the patient. If the patient has come because of a medical problem it is time to show the client what you have found in your examination. If the patient has come for routine vaccinations it is time to show the client any problems you have found during the basic well-patient examination. Show clients educational videos. Show them preserved samples of heartworms and roundworms, or of bladder stones, or of things you have removed from animals' stomachs, at appropriate times. Don't worry about offending the client with these "gross" samples. They will only be more motivated to work harder to prevent these awful parasites or medical conditions from affecting their pets.

This is the time to convert the intangible to the tangible. Anal sacs present one example to show and tell; just think of our client's little dog dragging its rear end up and down the white carpet and the pastel sofa. For anal sac treatment you need surgical gloves, an optical loop and sometimes a plastic apron. Follow anal sac expression with appropriate flushing and injection. If anal sac problems persist, do cultures and antimicrobial sensitivity testing. If those tests fail to uncover the problem, recommend anal sac removal. Dogs scooting their anus across the couch and carpet are legitimate concerns of our clients. Respect that concern. From the clients' viewpoint, successful resolution of scooting will be more impressive (more tangible) than your diagnosis and unsuccessful treatment of olgiodendrioglioma.

7. Give something.

Give the client some backup information: printed information concerning nutrition, obesity, dentistry, aging or something that pertains to the problem that brought the patient into your clinic. Do not let the client leave empty-handed.

He or she should have pertinent information about his or her pet, whether it is specific breed information, clinical information or perhaps a loaner tape for his VCR.

Clients feel more like they have received their money's worth if you can justify an injection to start the pet's treatment regimen. When a person has a purebred kitten, puppy or adult, send them home with information about their breed.

8. Compliment clients about their pets; reinforce their decisions.

Everyone's ego needs and enjoys occasional stroking. Compliment the client about his or her pet and about the good job he or she has done in caring for the animal. This pet is important to someone or these people would not be in your hospital. Every pet has something positive about it that you can compliment. It is cute, pretty, clean, sleek or fuzzy; or it is big or little, young or old, or healthy, or loved, or protective or sweet. There is something positive you can say.

If you have been listening, you will know what is most important about this pet to its owners. Many times the client feels guilty because the pet is ill, or overweight, or needs dentistry. You can bond them to your practice by being complimentary as well as helpful and sympathetic. Reinforce their actions by saying, "You sure are doing the right thing by bringing Fluffy in today."

9. Give clients the best options first.

Present the best treatment options first. Let the client decide if this treatment is too expensive. Don't be Dr. Gloom and Doom, unless the client refuses your advice which is given to assure comfort and wellness to the animal. Try to give them the "up" side of any prognosis or treatment. Say for an old dog: "Let's clean Spot's teeth so his breath will be sweet again and you'll allow him to sit in your lap again," rather than: "Spot is an older dog but I'm sure he'll come through a teeth cleaning okay." Always emphasize the benefits of treatments or procedures before you list the down sides, but *never, never* fail to tell clients about potential problems.

10. Close with ... "Have I answered all your questions?"

Post-visit surveys of physicians offices have shown that a primary frustration of clients is that doctors fail to answer all their questions. The same problem can sometimes be attributed to veterinarians. In addition, asking, "Have I answered all of your questions?" is a pleasant way to indicate the end of the exam.

According to the Krannert School of Business at Purdue University, there is a window of optimum time for clients to spend in the exam room. Less than 18 minutes could be too short and more than 32 minutes could be too long.

Seven steps to a higher recheck rate

by Dennis Cloud, DVM

Do you send your clients off with a vague reminder to "come back in three weeks," or to call if the animal "seems worse?" You'll please your clients, improve the medical care of their pets and boost your bottom line if you consistently follow this seven-step plan.

How many times have you told your clients:

- "If Rover isn't better in five days, call me."
- "When Fluffy finishes her medicine, let me know if she isn't better."
- "If that lump starts to grow, bring Sparky back in."

Most veterinarians are guilty of using these phrases, at least once in a while; but what many of us don't realize is that when we do, we're doing our patients and our clients a grave injustice. How? By making the client the doctor, and thus delegating to him or her *our* responsibility for evaluating the pet's health. The results can be fatal, or, at the very least, cost you the client's trust.

Seven-step recheck protocol

It is our responsibility not only to diagnose a patient's illness but to closely monitor its progress. To do so, the other doctors in my practice and I follow a seven-step protocol to encourage rechecks and, ultimately, to improve patient care. The steps are as follows:

1. Educate the client.

After you've completed the exam, explain to the client in detail the disease or condition of the animal, and the importance of rechecking the problem at a later date. Emphasize the negative consequences that can arise if the patient isn't monitored correctly.

2. Establish a convenient day of the week for scheduling the recheck.

Discuss with the client the day of the week that would be most convenient for him or her to come in for a recheck. You may want to start by suggesting that the client return on the same day of the week as the original visit.

3. Choose a specific date.

Using *your* calendar, which you should bring into the exam room with you, and which should include all of your upcoming professional obligations, work with the client to select a specific date for a recheck that is convenient for both of you. Be sure the client agrees to this date before you leave the exam room.

4. Fill out an appointment card.

While still in the exam room, fill out an appointment card in front of the client, noting on it the date of the pet's recheck.

5. Ask your receptionist to schedule an appointment time.

Accompany the client and pet to the front desk and ask your receptionist to schedule a convenient appointment time for the client on the chosen date. It's also a good idea to ask the receptionist to make sure he or she has the client's correct phone number for a reminder call. By conferring with the receptionist in the client's presence, you reinforce the importance of the recheck and boost the chances for compliance. Veterinarians who install computer terminals which can access appointment calendars in the exam room report a significant increase in recheck exams.

6. Send a reminder card.

If the recheck appointment is more than three weeks after the original visit, send the client a reminder card two weeks prior to the next appointment date.

7. Make a reminder phone call.

Make one reminder phone call. Ask your receptionist to call the client 24 hours prior to the recheck appointment, at which point any time conflicts that have arisen can be resolved.

Set a recheck goal. To successfully implement this program in your practice, you need to establish a recheck goal—then meet it with consistency. This goal should simply be the percentage of cases you believe you must recheck to provide adequate medical and surgical care to your patients. We believe we should achieve a minimum recheck rate of 38 percent of all of the cases we see. Incidentally, most of the other practices we've surveyed show recheck rates of only 10 to 12 percent.

How do you charge for rechecks? At our hospital, we charge $3 less for our rechecks than we do for our regular office call/exam. We've found, however, that our average transaction fee for recheck exams isn't significantly lower than our average charge per transaction.

Every step counts. Although I believe that maintaining a consistent recheck rate is the easiest part of this program, I realize that a seven-step protocol can be difficult to implement in a busy practice. If, however, every veterinarian in your practice follows all seven steps, you should see close to a 100 percent compliance rate. If you omit any of the steps, expect the percentage of rechecks to drop significantly. Total cooperation among doctors, staff and clients is essential to the success of this program.

Beyond the "10 Steps" and "Seven Steps"

In addition to the 10- and seven-step programs outlined above, it's important to keep the following specifics about communication in mind:

A. Rapport

- Talk about the client's special interest.
- Use the client's name.
- Smile.
- Be open and honest.

B. Empathy

- Touch.
- Pause.
- Ask questions.
- Be an "active listener."

This article originally appeared as "Seven Steps to a Higher Recheck Rate" in the April 1993 issue of *Veterinary Economics*. It is reprinted here by permission of the publisher.

Handling objections

by Ross D. Clark, DVM

Here's what professional sales people recommend we do when a client raises questions about a recommended treatment or recheck:

1. Don't assume that objections mean no.

Many people object automatically to anything new, unusual, unexpected or unbudgeted; it's called "posturing." The worst thing you can do for your patients, your hospital and your professional image is to accept a "no" without further discussion. If we take a "no" at face value and the patient leaves without proper medical attention, we will be the ones the client blames if the patient sickens, or even worse, dies. Clients will perceive us as not having cared enough to really explain the situation.

2. Look at objections as requests for further information.

If there hadn't been some concern on the client's part for the patient's health, he or she would not have consulted a professional. It is up to us to explain to our clients why we have recommended a specific procedure or course of treatment. By having further conversation, we can find out the reasons behind the "no." Give the client a detailed explanation of the recommended treatment or procedure. List all the benefits for the animal, and be sure to tell the client of any danger involved.

3. Restate objections.

Repeat the client's objections while agreeing that: "Yes, it is involved," or "Yes, I know how you feel" or "Yes, it can be expensive." Counter each objection with a positive benefit, such as, "It will extend your Fluffy's life," or "Fluffy will feel so much better and will have no more pain" or "Let me give you an estimate on how much it will cost."

4. Ask for agreement.

Once we have listened to the client, restated objections and stated benefits, we should ask the client for agreement. "How do you feel, Mrs. Jones?" Now it's time to ask him or her to agree with our professional opinion. We have told the client about the problem and about the solution. It is now up to him or her to make a decision from our positive presentation of the facts.

Training your staff to book more phone shoppers

by Marty Becker, DVM, owner of Compass Consulting and frequent lecturer and writer on the veterinary profession

Many veterinary hospitals have seen a dramatic increase in the number of phone shoppers. Why?

Because this is the value decade!

That's why we need to book more phone shoppers.

In an average practice, 15 to 20 percent of our clientele is lost each year through no fault of our own. Some people die, some pets die, others move away. Still others meet another veterinarian at church or a civic club. If we have 5,000 clients, that means we must replace 1,000 per year, or over three per day (most clinics aren't open 365 days per year) just to stay even!

The average client in a comprehensive practice spends well over $150 per year. So conservatively, if we book one more phone shopper per day for a year (250 days), that is $37,500 per year in income we will lose if we treat phone callers frivolously!

Perhaps most importantly, if you can convert telephone shoppers to clients, you can save pets' lives! Once they come in our doors, we can educate phone shoppers to make informed decisions concerning their pets' health and happiness. The number one killer of dogs in the United States is euthanasia—usually for no more reason than the owner's inability to handle minor problem behaviors. Therefore, it is critical to the lives of pets that we get people in the door so that we can educate them on optimizing their pets' health and help them with such life-saving matters as behavior training.

Tragically, few of us realize how many clients—and their pets—we unknowingly turn away from our practice every day due to the following problems:

- lack of skill,

- lack of knowledge,

- lack of training,

- lack of enthusiasm or

- lack of concern (indifference).

Does that sound like the hard sell? Consider it a must sell! Our goal is to sell them not everything they need, but only what they need for a happy, healthy pet. We realize that if we fail to get them in the door and get them to accept our professional recommendations and make all of the necessary buying decisions, there may be a premature or unnecessary death of a pet. We don't just lose the sale; we can lose a pet. It is a moral obligation we should not take lightly.

Who are we trying to book?

Our target market is:

- Women—According to the AVMA, 73 percent of the primary caregivers for pets are women.

- Baby-boomers—More than one in three Americans are baby-boomers.

- "Pet" owners—Owners of "pets," versus animals, consider their pets a part of the family.

There are basically three types of clients:

- The "caring" client—calls if the 30-pound cat misses a single meal!

- The "guilty" client—calls reluctantly after a lot of soul and wallet searching.

- The "new pet" client—"a lump of clay, ready to be molded" into a loving, responsible pet owner.

We can use many tools to get people to call our clinic so that we can "put fish in our pond." We can educate, arouse curiosity or identify a want or need by utilizing the following tools:

- Yellow pages;

- Flyers—e.g., one on house training pets;

- Referrals;

- Target people new to the area—over 60 percent own pets and over 75 percent need services within six months;

- Increase adoptions—Adopt out an average of two per day, 365 days per year;

- Reader boards—25,000 cars per day pass our clinic; and

- Classified ads (pet section)—critical to get them in before they go elsewhere.

Why do people phone shop?

Clients will phone shop on commodity items (goods and services that are routinely purchased and are often promoted on price alone) if they aren't bonded on the value you offer, if they are not emotionally and physically linked to the practitioner or the practice and if they feel like they can save a lot of money on the identical product or service. The key words here are "value," "a lot of money" and the "identical product or service!"

However, value means different things to different people, depending on their experiences, socioeconomic group and expectations. Trends also influence where people shop. In the "value decade," the trends are:

- To buy retail at wholesale prices;

- To wait until the prices go down; and

- Diminished loyalty.

Here's what you must offer to keep your clients from becoming phone shoppers:

- Value—Give enough benefits to justify the prices you charge. Create a higher buying decision ratio, as in, benefits/price = buying decision.

- Savings—Quote price at the lowest common denominator. For example, split out dollars for vaccine and exam; sponsor wellness programs.

- Extras—Make sure you offer value-added products and services. Vaccination warranty, *Bordetella* or bandannas, for example.

FAO Schwartz sells two-thirds private label products and one-third of their other products are priced competitively with Toys-R-Us.

I know this sounds like common sense to every practitioner, but I feel that if we concentrate even more on booking information calls and phone shoppers, we can dramatically increase our practice income, help pets be happier and healthier and even save pets' lives.

The bottom line is simple: we need more clients. Most of us are not operating anywhere near the capacity that would compromise the high level of customer and patient service we insist on delivering. And if your veterinary staff is on incentive pay, they all *want* to be busier!

Mystery shop

We frequently "mystery shop" our practice—by phone and in person—to objectively measure our customer service and quality control. The exercise has been a real eye opener. The staff knows that we do it and why we do it. We're striving to better serve pets and people. It is part of their performance review. We want to measure and evaluate everything from:

- How long did the phone ring before it was answered?

- What was the "tone level" of the pet counselor?

- Did we go through the "seven steps for booking phone shoppers" as outlined later in this chapter?

- Did the pet counselor give accurate information?

- Did we use the clients' and pets' names and refer to correct gender?

- Did we comfort the buying decision and thank them for calling?

With some very dedicated and caring employees with years of training, usually we run a very professional and efficient practice. But sometimes the staff and/or the systems break down and our machine sputters to a stop. Such was the case with our handling of the phones and phone shoppers before we changed our vision, systems, training and motivation.

The good thing about actually recording phone conversations is that you not only hear exactly what was said but can measure enthusiasm and feeling as well.

Recruiting help from my family, friends, neighbors and business contacts, I recorded about 25 conversations between "phone shoppers" and our hospital. The results were surprising although not very encouraging initially. But the experience made the entire hospital staff realize that we were:

- Not doing as well as we all thought (through indifference, being in a hurry, a lack of enthusiasm or inadequate training, etc.); and

- Not being pet advocates (spokespersons for a pet's best interests) as often or with as much dedication as we thought.

It was obvious that we didn't have to search beyond our own phone lines to find the increase in client visits we sought. Far too often, the receptionists were making serious and potentially life-threatening mistakes on the phone:

- Diagnosing over the phone. Not recommending or insisting strongly enough that clients come in to see the doctor, but rather agreeing that the client could watch the animal for a day or two first, try a home remedy, etc.;

- Giving inaccurate information; and

- Not asking for the appointment.

While mystery shopping, we were also charting the number of phone calls we received versus the number of appointments made. We found out that we were only booking about 25 percent of the phone shopping/information calls we were receiving! We needed to change our paradigm (our way of looking at and doing things). We had some "stale opinions" and "bad habits." We needed a "paradigm shift."

How and why change is necessary and correct

Send a "change message" message to your staff when needed. To send a "change message":

- Describe behavior specifically.

- Express the direct consequences to you (or the practice).

- Express change required.

- Express positive change = SUCCESS!!

- If necessary, repeat the previous steps several times.

- If still a problem, then negative consequences must be identified and exercised.

The action plan to increase our gross sales

We were now armed with facts (tapes of the phone calls and the graphs of calls versus appointments) and emotion (the realization that we weren't serving the best interests of pets or our clients). We were ready to make some significant changes to ensure that we would continue to improve in this vital area. We knew we needed "Smiles" and "Systems."

First the "smiles"

When someone at a business answers the phone, or when you walk in their front door, can you tell within milliseconds whether or not the person helping you is there because he or she "wants to be there" or "has to be there?" Yes! Within milliseconds!

Smiles (in person or on the phone) convey enthusiasm. They create energy that creates sales. "Smiles" increase your face value! And it's difficult to train it ... you've got to have it. To make sure, call all job applicants a couple of times at 7:30 a.m.! Sometimes they've faked enthusiasm to this point, and now you're testing their energy and "tone level" when they least expect it.

Then the "systems"

Here was our five-point plan for a better system:

- We all reviewed and critiqued the phone tapes.

- We obtained additional resource materials for telephone skills and set up additional training time for sales training, etc.—learning how to create a domino effect of "yes" answers.

- We put a seven-point telephone protocol by the phones and put a sticker that read, "Smile on the phone" on each phone.

- We agreed to intensify our mystery shopping efforts and appointment charting so that we would have more objective feedback. We agreed on how we would measure our performance, how often we would give feedback and, most importantly, what the consequences for success or failure would be.

- We agreed that our main motivation for this system was a "conscience for consequences" for pets and "celebrating and protecting the human-companion animal bond™."

We realized that in this business you don't just lose the sale ... you can lose the pet! And we also realized that it was an obligation to make the pet as happy and healthy as possible.

Seven steps to book phone shoppers

1. Start with an enthusiastic greeting.
2. Obtain information.
3. Sell the "personalized product."
4. Quote the benefits first ... then the price.
5. Ask for the appointment.
6. Reconfirm the details of the appointment.
7. Thank them for calling.

Review the following script for more detail and help in making this technique work for your practice.

Telephone script for vaccination price shoppers

Here is a script to handle inquiries about vaccination prices.
The following script assumes that you have already gone through
the first two steps to sales: (1) engaged the client in conversation
and (2) obtained information (diet, behavioral problems, vaccinations needed, etc.).

Client: I need to get my pet vaccinated. How much are
       the shots?

Pet Complex: Well Ms.____, your pet needs several vaccina-
       tions, including distemper-parvo-corona and a
       rabies vaccination. We want you to be aware of a
       couple of our exclusive programs so that you
       have enough information to make an informed
       decision.
       FIRST ... We stand behind the vaccines we use. If
       your pet gets any disease that we have vacci-
       nated it against during the entire year after
       having that booster administered at All Pet Com-
       plex, we will treat it and pick up the tab
       ourselves ... up to $1,000! This warranty is pro-
       vided at no cost to you. This remarkable
       cost-free warranty is made possible partly by the
       high quality of vaccines we use, and because
       each of our doctors gives the vaccine properly,
       ONLY after determining that your pet is healthy.
       SECOND ... We offer two vaccination programs
       that allow you to better match your budget and
       schedule with our recommendations for what
       your pet needs. We highly recommend that your
       pet gets an annual in-depth physical exam. This
       can help us catch many problems early on,
       before they become serious, cause unnecessary
       pain or expense ... or worse!
       Ms. ____ (client name), for ____ (pet's name) the

cost for the distemper-parvo-corona vaccine, rabies vaccine, comprehensive physical exam and professional consultation is $____.
Now, if you would prefer for ____ to have only a brief exam and vaccinations and you don't mind waiting in line sometimes, we offer "vaccination-value times:" Tuesday–Saturday from noon-2 p.m. and on Sunday from 10:30–noon. During these times we won't charge an examination fee, and the cost for ____'s vaccinations would be $____.
Which one would you prefer ... or do you have any questions? We have some openings today and on Saturday ... which one would you prefer?

The last part, I have italicized because it is critical. It gives the client a choice that makes it harder to just hang up and continue phone shopping!

Ten things *to* do:

- Use a proper greeting. "Thank you for calling. How may I direct your call?"

- Use the owner's name, pet's name and proper gender.

- Exude care and concern.

- Make strong recommendations, not suggestions.

- Give them reasons to come in.

- Communicate to the client the feeling that "they had me in mind when they created these goods and services."

- Under-promise and over-deliver.

- Be knowledgeable; but don't be afraid to say, "I don't know—but I'll find out."

- Have a "conscience for consequences."

- Answer every question with a product, a service or TLC.

Four things *not* to do...

- Treat a caller like just another shopper.

- Make the owner feel stupid for being concerned or having called.

- Diagnose over the phone.

- Fail to give the caller your undivided attention and concern.

We don't need to worry about "the competition" when trying to figure out how to "jump-start" our own practice and make it thrive. You've heard the old saying, "What gets measured gets done?" Well, it's true. But more importantly, in this case we realized that our indifference and our lack of enthusiasm, training and skill were directly or indirectly causing the unnecessary or premature death of pets. It was a sobering finding.

The number of phone contacts that we convert to appointments has tripled. Business is up! All this time, the increased business we sought was right under our noses ... the right words just needed to come out of our mouths. It has been several years since we started this program, and we are still experiencing great results!

Advertising your practice

by Ross D. Clark, DVM

Advertising:
"Boy meets girl, tells girl how wonderful he is..."

Promotion:
"Boy meets girl, tells girl how wonderful she is..."

Marketing:
"Boy meets girl, researches her hobbies and interests, directs his attention to those areas..."

Public Relations ("reputation management"):
"Girl hears from others how wonderful boy is..."

> *Hill & Knowlton Ad Agency,*
> *Purina-ProPlan Marketing Seminar for*
> *Industry Leaders, January 1991.*

> *"Half the money I spend on advertising is wasted, and the trouble is, I don't know which half."*
>
> *Lord Leverhulme*

Advertising is the engine that powers commerce. Veterinarians are just becoming comfortable with the word "marketing," and the idea of "advertising" can still be disconcerting even now, in the mid '90s. But by the turn of the century, advertising will be commonplace in the veterinary marketplace.

I can remember when established veterinarians frowned on colleagues who sent postcard reminders, although first-class letters were somewhat acceptable. Working with pet stores and breeders was considered prostitution of the profession.

The facts about advertising:

- Advertising is expensive.
- Advertising is not an exact science.

Advertising often asks us to change, leave our comfort zone for something new and improved. But it can also ask us not to change. It can tell us, "You did the right thing."

The statement, "Our company has been the community leader for 30 years," for instance, suggests that our clientele should not risk the unknown of a new clinic with inexperienced veterinarians and green staff members.

Effective advertising tries to convince the consumer that your veterinary hospital is the way to go. It reminds clients and potential clients of your presence in the community and urges action to properly protect and care for their treasured pets. Effective advertising clearly identifies your location and tells clients how to get there. It also reaffirms the clients' notion that your clinic is one of the best and many other clients like and use your services. You have a wide array of choices to create effective advertising, including:

Point-of-purchase

The point-of-purchase option is a good choice because it can change a $60 visit into an $80 visit with very little extra effort. Point-of-purchase promotions provide convenience to your clients. The only downside is the competition for space. If you have plenty of space, point-of-purchase advertising makes sense.

Radio

Radio can be targeted to a specific age group and income level; and, because it is less expensive than television, you can purchase a higher frequency advertising. It should be used to support your image and remind the community of your presence. Rich Cohn of Tulsa Z104.5 counsels his clients to distance themselves from the business and see things objectively through the clients' eyes. Reduce marketing strategies to a simple few.

- Know what makes the business and its products or services unique.

- Test the marketing message.

- Repeat, repeat, repeat.

Business owners are often too content to accept what's important to them as what's important to their clients. Repetition is important in radio because listeners tune in and out, do errands and occasionally stop paying attention. If you don't have the attention of listeners within five seconds, your ad loses effectiveness. Mention your name at least five times in a 30-second spot. Use simple straightforward sentences. Try your ad on a 12-year-old. If he or she doesn't understand it, it's probably too complicated.

Television

Television is regarded as a good choice for giant companies wanting to reach the entire trade area. Television is too expensive for most practices with fewer than 10 veterinarians. For large "multiple-practice" practices in large metropolitan areas, television sometimes may be cost-effective. For now, television is only feasible for the largest operations.

Newspapers

The large city newspapers are much like television—covering too much distance and far too many people to be cost effective. Local or community newspapers can be somewhat effective.

Outdoor billboards

Outdoor billboards can reach a large audience with geographic flexibility. Billboards are viewed repeatedly by a regular audience, creating great brand-name recognition. They work for you 24 hours a day, seven days a week. Their main limitation is the requirement for very simple, short messages.

Indoor billboards

Indoor billboards at airport terminals deliver the high-income families and business executives that we desire as "top flight" clients. Airports are a good place to market your boarding.

Direct mail

Direct mail should probably be our advertising and marketing medium of choice. We should completely develop our direct-mail programs such as sending at least three reminders plus special newsletters to retired Greyhound owners, German Shepherd owners, Dalmatian owners, Scottish Fold owners and the like. Direct mail is a precision tool for reaching the persons most likely to utilize veterinary services.

Telephone directories and yellow pages

The yellow pages directory is not a bad choice. It is the only advertising medium where you have buyers seeking sellers. Yellow pages are there when a potential client is actually making that decision to call a veterinarian. Yellow pages are opened 24 hours a day and probably are a cost-effective method of advertising our services.

Yellow-page consultants recommend that you include as much copy as you can comfortably fit in the space you can afford. Russell Marketing Research conducted a study in which "copy-heavy" ads drew more response by a two-to-one ratio Use convincing copy to persuade prospective clients that you are experienced and reliable.

The larger the ad, the more information you can convey. Include color when you can. That draws attention to your ad. Include your logo and company name. Let people know where they can find your hospital.

Guidelines for yellow page advertisers:

- Don't use fine-line artwork that won't reproduce well on soft yellow newsprint.

- Do what you can to have a memorable phone number.

- Don't use dumb cartoons, puns, "unclever" slogans or your children's pictures. People looking in the yellow pages are hot buyers looking for a professional source.

- Use strong borders—the blackest allowed. Lump type into smaller areas to give emphasis to those areas and keep type away from the border. The reader's eye will go to your ad.

- Line illustrations usually reproduce better than photographs, but don't clown. Cartoons are for the comic strips, not the yellow pages.

- Do not be too sharp. The serious buyer resents smugness. Copy should be warm but businesslike.

- Don't be afraid of long copy. Research shows that long copy outpulls short copy in the yellow pages.

National yellow pages study findings*:

- Yellow pages are the medium most often used when looking for veterinary services.

- Seventy percent of those who look for a veterinarian through the yellow pages are women.

- Thirty-four percent of those who shop the yellow pages for veterinary services have no hospital in mind.

- Almost half (49 percent) of those who shop the yellow pages "shop around" and look at more than one listing.

- Ninety percent of those who turn to the yellow pages for veterinary services make a call.

*from *AAHA Trends*, December 1994–January 1995

Advertising Research Corporation says:

- As the ad size increases, selection levels increase.

- Doubling ad size does not double selection levels.

- Users seem to prefer "display" ads.

- "Cluttered" headings have less impact.

- Stepping up your ad under a less cluttered heading brings the greatest return.

- Most users start looking at the first or second page of the yellow pages listings.

- Quarter-page ads show a decrease in selection as they appear closer to the front of the listing.

- Half-page ads out-perform quarter-page ads.

- "Shoppers" respond more to the size of the ads than do directional users (those with a veterinarian in mind).

- Advertisers with low public profiles see the greatest rise in calls by increasing ad size.

AdLab* tips

AdLab, a company that specializes in yellow pages, recommends taking the following steps to make more money from advertising in that medium.

First, understand what is important to your prospective customers or clients, so you can choose the right theme.

Second, understand the process that most prospects go through, so your ad gets through their screening. Even when someone makes a judgment call with insufficient information, he or she will try to make it rationally. They won't just flip a coin. How do you make their "cut?"

Consider the following points:

- Yellow pages advertising is "direct response" advertising.

- The majority of people who turn to the yellow pages call one or more of the advertisers.

- Recognition and recall advertising is the most common.

- The yellow pages should make users call you instead of your competition.

- The ad must be big enough to explain your business.

- More information equals more calls ... information is more important than "white" space in the yellow pages.

- If yours is already the biggest veterinary ad, however, you don't need to go up in size, even if your yellow pages representative tells you that "bigger is better."

*AdLab specializes in effective yellow page ads. They can be reached by writing, faxing or calling: Robert H. Breinholt, Ph.D., 2880 South Main St., Salt Lake City, UT 84115; phone: (800) 221-0254; (801) 486-2348; (801) 486-2380.

- Ask yourself, "Am I making money on my current ad?
- Color attracts readers (shoppers, customers, clients).

Five steps to getting the call:

1. Get their attention with pictures of happy, smiling and attractive people enjoying the benefits of your services.

2. Gain their interest with a thematic headline. To pick your theme, first understand what is important to your clients. Do not put your hospital name at the top of the ad page, put benefits first. Determine the most common problems clients might be trying to solve—itching and scratching, for instance—and put *that* at the top.

3. Give them information: This should be the "body" of the ad copy—the more information, the more calls.

4. Build conviction.

5. Close the ad with "call us soon" instead of the more demanding "call us first."

The best single step you can take to make your yellow page advertising make more money is "get some professional help."

Budgeting for advertising

Advertising and marketing costs are completely controllable expenses. That you have decided to read this chapter suggests that you feel either a need to attract new clients or a need for exposure to keep top-of-the-mind awareness among your clients.

What you would like to invest and what you can afford to invest in advertising are rarely the same. Spending too much may be an obvious and repugnant display of extravagance; however, spending too little can be just as hardheaded and overly conservative in today's marketplace.

The most widely used method of establishing an advertising budget is to base it on a percentage of gross sales. There is one main pitfall of using profits as a base. If you experience a period in which profits are low, it may or may not be because of too much or too little advertising. You in fact may objectively and correctly determine a need for additional advertising during low-profit times. In the short term, cutting advertising budgets can result in improved profits but may not be the best solution.

What is the right percentage?

The typical small-animal hospital with two veterinarians spends about one percent of its gross on advertising, marketing and promotion when you include yellow pages and business section listings. These averages are not gospel. As consolidation of our profession progresses, I suspect this percentage will become larger. McDonald's spends four to five percent on its marketing and advertising program, and Radio Shack has been known to spend up to nine percent of gross sales.

The Guerrilla Marketing Handbook (Boston: Houghton Mifflin, 1994) recommends 10 percent as a rule of thumb. It says that some businesses like cigarettes and perfume require more. I believe businesses spending 10 percent or more of gross on marketing and advertising must have a much better mark up than we do in veterinary medicine.

You can calculate your advertising budget based on past gross, projected gross or a combination of the two. Our practice currently spends two percent on marketing, promotion, yellow pages, public relations and other advertising. I think five percent would be too high and one percent too low for our Tulsa market.

Source:

Lewis, H. G. *How to Make Your Advertising Twice as Effective at Half the Cost.* Chicago: Dartnell Corporation, 1987.

Technician Power: Eight steps to a great exam-room visit

By Ross D. Clark, DVM

Medical protocols are important, but the way you approach *humans* in the exam room will either bond clients to your practice—or send them packing. Technicians can follow these eight steps to assure an office visit everyone will enjoy.

Medical procedures may be your strong point, but veterinary personnel aren't using their skills to full advantage if they don't think about the human side of veterinary medicine every day. As the first medical professional to talk to clients, technicians set the tone for the visit, which gives them the opportunity and the responsibility to bond clients to the hospital.

As a veterinary technician, each time you enter an exam room, you can make the difference between a client who is on the defensive when the doctor enters and a client who is ready to accept advice and further service from professionals who obviously care about him or her and the pet. I've heard of clients who want to change veterinarians—but don't because they wouldn't dream of leaving the caring and professional staff. To fine-tune your personal presentation, follow these steps:

1. Present yourself as a medical professional.

What reassures you when you visit your doctor? The same approach will reassure your clients:

- Wear an appropriate uniform and a name badge. These details send a strong professional message.

- Introduce yourself and shake hands with the clients as soon as you enter the exam room. Come out from behind the exam table to greet them, and keep in mind that many clients are apprehensive and deeply concerned about their pets' well-being.

• Wash your hands in the exam room or walk in drying your hands.

• Your body language communicates volumes, in fact, communication experts say that as much as 65 percent of communication is nonverbal. When you introduce yourself, concentrate on your tone of voice, posture and eye contact to send clients the message that you're capable, knowledgeable, confident and caring.

• Try to use your name and the client's name at least three times during the visit. Doing so helps create a friendly and professional atmosphere. And, after you see a client for a number of visits, ask him or her to use your first name. People love to do business with a friend, and you want them to look forward to seeing you.

2. Build confidence while you take a brief history and note problems for the doctor to check.

The pets you see are cherished companions and their acceptance of you is important to their owners. By talking to the client and touching the pet, you build the client's confidence—and help allay the animal's fears. Pet owners want you to like their pets.

In fact, clients must feel that their animals' well-being is your hospital's most important function. When I ask clients why they switched hospitals, many tell me they felt the staff didn't like Dobermans or cats or their dog in particular. Their reason? The doctor and technician spent very little time touching or talking to the pet.

To send a positive message, touch the animal and talk to both pet and owner as you do your work. It's up to you to instill confidence in them!

3. Reinforce the client's opinion of you as a medical professional.

The exam-room duties of technicians vary from hospital to hospital, but whatever your role, keep the client apprised of what you're doing and speak in quiet tones that soothe the animal. If the patient is calm and friendly, do all of the work in the exam room—clients like to see what they're paying for. The more they see you do, the higher the perceived value of the services.

If the pet seems highly irritable, ask the owner's permission to remove the animal to a treatment room. I've witnessed a few disasters in which clients, technicians and doctors were soiled with blood, feces, and urine trying to trim a Chihuahua's toenails in the exam room. I'm sure such scenes don't help our professional image.

Of course, removing a pet from the owner can be a delicate matter. Be sure the client approves. Ask the client to reassure the pet and, if possible, to hand the animal to you so the patient knows the owner approves of you.

4. Show and tell.

The next step is to offer the client information on the future good health of the patient. For example, if the client brought the pet in for routine vaccinations, mention any problems you found during the basic well-pet examination and discuss preventive care.

It's also a good idea to show clients educational videos and preserved samples of heartworms, roundworms or bladder stones. Don't worry about offending them with these "gross" samples. By seeing them firsthand, they'll only be more motivated to prevent these awful parasites or conditions from harming their cherished pets. Your professional expertise can help make intangible medical threats tangible to your clients.

5. Provide educational materials.

Don't let clients go home empty-handed! Hand each pet owner printed information on nutrition, obesity, dentistry, aging or any other subject that pertains to the problem that brought the patient to your clinic. It's information they need to maintain the long-term health and happiness of the pet.

In my clinic, we send owners of purebreds home with a colorful folder that includes information on each animal's breed. You might create and offer similar folders for other clients, including new clients and exotic pet owners.

Handouts on preventive care and common medical problems are available from manufacturers or for purchase from such organizations as the American Animal Hospital Association (P.O. Box 150899, Denver, CO 80215; phone: 303-986-2800; fax: 303-986-1700).

6. Compliment the client and reinforce his or her decision to own a pet.

Everyone needs and enjoys an occasional ego stroking. Compliment clients on their pets and the good job they do caring for them. Every pet deserves a compliment: Perhaps it's pretty, clean, fuzzy, big, little, young, old, healthy, protective or sweet. There's usually something positive you can say that shows you care and understand this pet's importance. If you listen carefully, the owner will likely tell you why the pet is so important.

Keep in mind that clients may feel guilty because the pet is overweight, ill or needs dentistry. Being complimentary, helpful, and sympathetic helps make them more comfortable—and bonds them to your practice. Tell clients you know how easy it is to run out of time in a busy life. If you offer such services, tell them about early drop-offs, pick-up or deliveries. Reinforce the visit by saying, "You did the right thing bringing Fluffy in today."

7. Prepare for the veterinarian.

Prepare vaccines and any equipment needed to help the doctor be efficient while in the exam room. In some hospitals, one doctor and one technician work together throughout the day as a "care pair." During slow times, the technician stocks the exam rooms with necessary equipment, medicates hospitalized patients, makes call-backs on the previous day's patients or prepares medications for pets to be dismissed that day. Other hospitals find it more efficient for a pool of technicians to assist the doctors as needed.

8. Be each client's advocate as he or she prepares to depart.

Assist your clients—whose hands are likely to be full of leashes, printed materials and products (ideally placed in a logo-imprinted bag)—to the discharge area. Depending on your clinic set-up, introduce clients to the cashier or reintroduce them to the receptionist. Help them make an appointment for their next visit or recheck. And help them to the car if they need it. Good service is always welcome and remembered warmly.

Today, there's hardly a town of any size that doesn't offer a choice of veterinarians. The client in your exam room chose your clinic, and you are first in line to impress him or her with the caring medical professionals in your hospital. It's important to confer with the doctor before you make major changes in your exam-room protocol, but chances are he or she will applaud your desire to bond clients and their pets to your practice.

Chapter 5:
Medical Records

by Thomas E. Catanzaro, DVM, MHA, Dipl. American College
of Healthcare Executives

Medical records for quality and profit

As the Director of Hospital Services at American Animal
Hospital Association (AAHA) from 1988 to 1991, I was very
involved with the evolution of the "standards" as well as the medical record requirements. Our profession is in transition. In
previous decades, AAHA only required legible records; but now,
continuity of care and quality of care have become the standard.
Our consulting team and AAHA committees developed sample
forms and formats, which were then offered to the profession to
assist in upgrading the quality of the forensic and health-care
documentation.

When comparing hard-copy medical records to computerized
record keeping, I believe that our first goal should be to meet the
health-care delivery standards of the veterinary profession.
Automation goals of most vendors are focused on the money.

They start at the end, the invoice. Although evolutionary changes have occurred in veterinary medical software programs to provide more "bells and whistles," what we still need is veterinary medical software with a database driven from the progress notes, not the invoice.

As such, I share my current prejudices and bias concerning electronic data processing (EDP) and quality health care.

- *Computers* are great for client relations, tracking income centers and even handling accounts payable.

- *Hard-copy medical records* are the means of professional communications between providers. Medical records ensure continuity of quality care.

  a) The Problem Oriented Medical Record (POMR) is a documentation requirement which is here to stay. This is what defeats lawyers in court!

  b) Forms can be individualized for each practice and its veterinarians. There is no single standard of "completeness." You should create forms that will enhance your efforts as a dedicated health-care provider. Do not let forms become too detailed and cumbersome. Design your forms for convenient page turning. (I prefer head-to-foot printing so I can turn up the page and keep writing on the back without undoing the prong.)

  c) Forms going home with clients *must* display your practice logo and phone number.

  d) Forms being used in-house require only client and patient names.

"Facts of life"

Having visited over 800 veterinary hospitals, I have developed a strong personal belief in veterinarians as a health-care delivery team rather than just primary providers. Through my observations, I have developed what I call the "facts of life."

- Good medical records increase continuity of patient care. I have seen some practices able to achieve 89 percent client compliance with full preventative services on the first visit and other practices that maintained current vaccination status within five percent of the initial-visit vaccination status.

- Low rates of return ("pets not seen in over 24 months") can be partially attributed to not recording health statistics on "other" pets in a multiple-pet household at the time one pet is brought in.

- Most "apparent" violations of internal policy or quality patient care are actually failures in the documentation process. These "failures" in documentation often led to internal control problems, liability and forensic concerns, embarrassment of the practice or client or a reduced value per pet seen. Failures in documentation reduce the ability of medical records to provide continuity of care as well as decrease the liquidity of the practice.

Your head receptionist should be responsible for consolidating medical records. When I hear a receptionist say, "that part of the medical record is not my concern," I know there is a problem.

The world of veterinary health care is going to the standard medical record folder, with hanging pocket systems (ANCOM, Profiles, etc.) or terminal-digit medical record file folders on open shelves. Any 5x7 note card system requires re-evaluation. Good medical records have a litigation protection value. Legal problems have ensued from incidents such as:

- performing tumor surgery without recorded client permission;

- admitting pets without noting action;

- prescribing medication without recorded reason;

- continuing furosemide treatment of cardiac dysfunction patients without recorded diagnostics or follow-up;

- performing surgery without recorded reason;

- not recording dental status, weight, temperature, pulse and respiration for each visit by the same pet;

- performing surgery without presurgical assessments;

- performing treatments without recorded reasons;

- providing in-patient care without vaccinations or client waiver;

- discharging patients without a discharge plan;

- contradicting records or ignoring records in successive entries; and

- recording ambiguous statements, such as "shots current" with no approximate date given.

To help avoid litigation:

- Record everything that is done, at the time it is done. Even a complimentary nail trim during surgery should be recorded, since any adverse sequelae might be cause for litigation or complaint. Most practice acts do not let veterinarians "hide" their health-care delivery.

- Charge for everything that is done, even if you have to spread expenses out over a period of time to make payment easier for the client.

- Don't set yourself up for failure by stating there isn't enough time to document quality veterinary health-care delivery.

Putting it together

Medical documents can be good for the practice only if they are used as designed, which has seldom been the case in records audited.

Summary forms include procedure tracking sheets, new client forms, and patient data cover sheet.

Progress notes forms are for recording care, needs and most importantly, client desires, waivers and deferrals. Medical record progress notes are the cornerstone of any health-care delivery program. They substantiate the charge sheet, and also allow another veterinarian in the practice to follow a case and ensure continuity of care.

Ten-step program

This program of recording an office visit from door (entrance) to door (exit) has proved to be effective in the search for veterinary excellence, in the quest for higher client transactions and for increased protection from litigation.

1. The client and pet arrive through the clearly marked entrance and are greeted by smiling faces. (The first always happens; the latter is often variable.)

2. After pleasant salutation with the client, the pet is immediately weighed. If the client is new, the New Patient/Client Form is initiated.

3. The receptionist initiates a procedure tracking sheet and patient progress notes. On the progress notes, the receptionist enters the date followed by the patient's problem in the client's own words.

    The receptionist should *not* enter interpretations such as "check skin" or "check ears." After the presenting complaint, he or she writes a box ☐; e.g., "rear smells ☐."

4. The second entry to be made by the receptionist concerns past-due protective health care. The entry method can be cryptic and simplified to meet practice needs. For example, he or she might say, "I notice that Spot appears past due for some preventive health care. I have made a note so our technician (or doctor) will remember to discuss this with you." But the notes would look something like: "RV ☐, dhppc ☐," etc. to indicate past due vaccinations

5. The technician then moves the client and patient from the reception area to an exam room and finishes the interview required for the new patient/client sheet, which is an exam room function, not a reception area function. The technician is responsible for initiating the physical examination checkup card, obtaining a history, performing a wellness exam and recording his or her findings on the report card. The technician's notes should be simple entries, such as "temp 105.3 ☐, dental 2+ ☐, enlarged l.n. R shoulder ☐," etc. The technician should also identify other animals in the household and enter or update their medical histories.

6. The veterinarian should read the technician's notes before entering the room. Then after examining the patient, he or she adds any exam or history factors important to the current or future continuity of care, including use of stickers or pictures (available through PETCOM, AAHA, etc.). Entries need to be linked with patient advocacy, client-centered service and client bonding to the practice for continuity of care and better profit. Once this is done, the veterinarian enters the assessment(s).

The assessment needs to start with the client's initial concern but can take many forms. The simplest signalment is the rule out (R/O). R/O is ONLY what we tell the client we are planning to treat for. It supports the medicine or action plan which follows. R/O is **NOT** a differential diagnosis. While "dx" (tentative diagnosis) and "ddx" (differential diagnosis), and "A" is assessment of the above information, none of these three signalments (dx, ddx, A) has proved to be forensically safe. Only R/O has not yet been litigated to the detriment of the health-care provider.

When these assessments or R/O need to be followed, they should appear on the patient data cover sheet (summary cover sheet problem list), with an entered date that matches the progress notes. Eventually, most every problem list entry should also achieve a resolved date to ensure continuity of care.

The assessment (R/O) can show "symptomatic tx" and the treatment can show the drug and full directions (including the strength, dose, frequency of treatment, duration of medication use, etc.).

It is important to clearly record what the client was told and how the client responded. A simple code system should be used. I use a box (☐) to denote a "need" on the progress notes (e.g., X-ray ☐ or CBC ☐) and a code to enter the client's response in the box.

Suggested codes include:

"W" = waived/refused by client

"D" = deferred by client or doctor until later time

"A" = appointment to be made

"X" = did it!

"+" = positive finding

"-" = negative finding

"na"= not applicable at this time

After the recommended procedure is done, an "X" is added, with the progress notes showing the findings (e.g., "X-ray⚀ABD VD & LAT⚀congestion R apical lobe.")

Subsequent treatment plans are established, reflecting the decisions based on the clinical findings (and stated in a modified R/O). All previous boxes need to be filled in, especially when ensuring the presenting complaint/concern has been solved in the client's mind.

After the doctor enters the medicines and procedures desired, then the statement, "Let's review what we've done today" is an excellent method of moving to the patient data cover sheet (pink and blue paper can be used to denote gender) and ensuring that the client understands what has occurred. This summary sheet uses the same codes as the progress notes, in the "checkerboard square" after every "wellness care" item.

7. The three *"R"s* (recheck/remind/recall) need to be addressed by the attending veterinarian to close out every last entry for each patient record. Client education needs to occur at this time also, either by the doctor or technician.

The technician draws and labels the medicines, administers the first dose with the client as a client training technique, ensures the client has the appropriate handouts and understands their importance, verifies all procedures have been circled on the tracking sheet, and all the boxes ☐ on the progress notes have been closed with an entry, then escorts the client and patient to discharge.

The three "R"s (recheck, recall, and reminder) are an important part of the waiver W̲ and deferral D̲ action. They are the subsequent visit desires and were introduced by Dr. Ross Clark in the early 1980s. They are part of this client communication process and are located at the top or bottom of the procedure tracking form. The next contact expectation must be established BEFORE the client departs, in order to achieve the best compliance and return rates. If the memory jogs are already on the tracking sheet, then all that is required is for the veterinarian(s) to use the form as designed. No animal should ever leave any practice facility without being in at least one of the three "R" categories, and most pets will likely be in multiple reminder categories.

8. While the doctor is finishing up, the technician has time to set up another client/patient in another exam room. The veterinarian will then have another client ready and can then move directly to the next exam room.

9. Clients should not be allowed to depart while there is still an empty ☐ indicating that health-care action is still needed. Even without the "box system," NO medical record should ever be filed if it is missing any of the following key elements:

    • Client complaint

    • Vaccination/preventive health update

    • Assessment(s)

    • Full medical directions

    • At least one of the three "Rs"

    • The doctor should not be allowed to depart for the day until all medical records are completed. Records should not be kept out of the system overnight because tomorrow has no more time than today.

10. Upon completion of the client's visit, the receptionist should use the procedure tracking sheet (circle sheet) as the source document for making computer entries, allowing a generated receipt (internal controls), and tracking of the three "Rs."

Some receptionists have convinced their veterinarians to get the charge sheet printed in red ink, so the doctor can continue to use black or blue-black ink, just like in the medical records, and the marks will show up easier.

Please consider that the circle sheet could also be used for updating any off-line computer database for ownership evaluation, for monitoring doctor efficiency, or initiating peer review. If an item is not needed in the computer, it does not need to be on the tracking sheet; it should be in the medical record if it pertains to health-care delivery.

Bear in mind that even within the 10 steps for medical record keeping, there are many alternatives. For example, the use of mega-stamp or the break-and-stick labels (eyes, dermatology, dental, physical, euthanasia, surgical summary, UA, etc.) to illustrate the observations may reduce the number of different forms required.

Tips for improving medical record keeping

The appointment system must match the doctor's style; but inversely, the doctor's style must match the practice economics. Options include the variable-length appointment program, new appointment logs, and the retraining of veterinarians to refer patients to themselves for inpatient care rather than defeating the appointment log.

You should write things only once in the progress notes; whenever possible. The plan can show the specific medication and strength while the treatment shows the amount, frequency and duration of use.

The alternatives provided to the client must be stated as "needs," for the animal. The terms "should" or "recommend" or "it would be best that" do not belong in health-care delivery; the Practice Act specifically states doctors can *only* provide "needed care" to a patient.

All health care initially needs to be based on the expectation for positive client action now or later. Offering "yes or no" choices has to stop. As patient advocates, veterinarians should instead offer their clients two ways to say "yes."

The only thing we really "sell" in veterinary health care is peace of mind; the client is allowed to "buy" what they feel they want at that point in time. The hard sell does not work in health care. If the client "can't afford it," pursue what that phrase means on that day ... payday may be tomorrow or the checkbook may have been left at home.

If the client declines the best level of care for the pet, record it in the book, defer (D) the care, try an acceptable alternative for a few days and attempt to schedule a recheck.

Supplemental forms may be useful for facilitating program delivery, but are counterproductive if used to replace talking to clients. Useful supplemental forms include:

- *Preanesthetic releases* with laboratory test waivers have proved to be profitable and a benefit to the patient. If phrased as a waiver (every client's right), most clients will accept the appropriate level of care.

- *Discharge forms* are memory jogs and client aids, but should not replace verbal communication. Like brochures, they are provided to the client "for later use at home" *after* a full discussion has transpired.

As I mentioned before, forms can assist programs; but it requires caring and concerned individuals to make the program work within any practice.

The *perception* of quality care is communicated in the exam room as well as during the hundreds of other personal encounters a client has with the doctor and staff during every visit. It does not matter to most clients what your grades were, how many years you went to school or what kind of equipment you have. They want to know that you believe that the care you offer is the best available. This is strictly a factor of communication. It is the staff and doctor pride that is perceived as quality. Pursue *pride* as the input of health care, and the outcome will be beneficial to the practice as well as the client and patient.

Empower key managers and veterinarians, with the help of the paraprofessional staff, to seek methods to streamline data collection efforts so that the clients or staff only have *to write the support data once.*

If the "secret codes" at the top of the patient data form are adopted, they need to be understood by each staff member without being written. These can be dangers, reminders or other items a practice does not want written "in the clear" for a client to read. The client education handouts key needs to be written and available, with a date of the most current handout reference for each number, if they are listed on any medical form.

The "checkerboard square" on the patient data cover sheet is the handwritten back-up to the computer system as well as a quick cross reference for other animals in the household, so the habits for completion need to be established. These are memory jogs that make the health-care review process complete and comprehensive; they also insure that an exit summary is provided to each client by the doctor so they will realize the value(s) their pet just received from the veterinarian or staff.

Patient advocacy

Veterinary staff need to be convinced that patient advocacy means promoting what's best for the patient *and* the client. That includes grief counseling, offering compassion and letting clients make their own decisions, as well as completely explaining the quality care the pet just received. The AAHA pet loss videotape series and the AAHA children's books elaborate on this theme.

A true patient advocate will tell the owner what is needed and explain the pros and cons. Medical records of patient advocacy will reflect veterinarian-deferred care, client waiver of animal rights and patient care above the "average" levels seen in the USA.

Internal marketing and patient advocacy are often confused, and that is okay. Marketing in a professional setting has three parts.

- Make the client aware of pre-existing needs of the animal. (This is also patient advocacy.)

- Offer the client relief from the concerns about the needs by offering a service that the profession and your practice can now fulfill. (This is internal marketing.)

- Give the client two choices to meet the animal's needs (or the doctor's needs) then be quiet—the first person to talk loses. (This is smart business.)

Peer review

The use of a "peer review system" has been suggested as a means of professional staff development. This is the next level of quality that needs to be addressed in veterinary health-care delivery. It is based on random cases being reviewed for content, treatment modalities, forensic concerns and continuity of care. It has been proven to be so essential in human health care that the Joint Commission for the Accreditation of Health-care Organizations now mandates such a program as a prerequisite for qualification for third-party reimbursements.

To initiate peer review within your own office, first establish a meeting time for all doctors. Have a receptionist select two in-patient and two out-patient records per doctor per month. Evaluate the cases in terms of the following questions:

- Can I follow this case without embarrassing the practice?

- Can I address the client without embarrassing myself, the other doctor or the client?

- Am I willing to stand up in a group of peers and state, from what was written, that the animal got the best care possible?

Any rationalization or justification is allowed by the doctor of record, but it must be understood that these types of "reasons/ excuses" are just indicators of inadequate medical records and probably inadequate health-care delivery.

The system discussed above works, but so do others. Start documenting the quality of health care that is being delivered; record the waivers and deferrals. By giving the client the right to say yes or no, 75 percent will say yes. Regardless, the health-care documentation system adopted needs to meet the practice philosophy.

The system selected needs to be integrated and contemporary. The alternatives are many, but what is most important is that clear practice expectations are needed and someone needs to make that happen! Be that someone in your practice; start doing it now!

Computerized medical records:
A consultant's observations

The following observations are the result of a single sit-down brainstorm session. It is only a starting point, and needs interactive development to even be considered usable.

While the computer has become the primary client relations tool, the medical record needs to be the cornerstone of the continuity of patient care, whether it is done by computer or on paper. The invoicing and reminders, while critical to the business of veterinary practice, are secondary to this health-care requirement.

Computerized medical records are based on a data base where a single medical record entry drives multiple retrieval systems, from inventory adjustments and invoicing to prescriptions and treatment plans.

In reality, multiple pieces of information drive the system. Client concern drives the examination protocol and diagnostic tests. The case assessment drives the treatment plan and dispensing actions. The follow-up expectations, as well as client waivers, deferrals and acceptances, reflect the official veterinary medical agreements made with the steward of the animal for the health-care treatment for the patient.

Reality test: If this data base "system" really exists, I could do the following query (although it may require multiple queries to get the classifications delineated, the original input would be from the single entry progress notes):

Retrieve all bilateral canine otitis externa cases seen in the past eight months, compare treatment results and return rates for those treated with (1) Panolog®, (2) Tresaderm®, (3) Mitox™ or (4) Otomax®, and show the average total cost and average client transaction income associated with each treatment modality.

Some problems with computer records:

- **Shortcuts to follow-up exams.** The POMR format is the accepted level of competency in veterinary medical records. It is based on four elements: Subjective (History), Objective (Exam), Assessment (what are we treating) and Plan (here is what we can do); thus, the acronyms "SOAP" or "HEAP." Current computer software bypasses some aspects of this exam format on follow-up visits (which constitute 10 to 30 percent of our caseload). When an assessment is initially made and entered into the "Master Problem List" of the computer, a number is assigned. On return visits for the same problem, the computer skips over the SOA or HEA portion of the record and allows the provider to go directly to the new/revised/modified treatment plan.

- **Bypass of critical information.** There are certain critical elements of information required in the progress notes of the medical records. Industry standards are set by AAHA and universities. They are modified by the AVMA trust agents who settle medical record litigation out of court. Required information includes:

  a) Patient specific medical records (client-patient)

  b) Date of presentation

  c) Client concerns (chief complaint) at presentation

  d) Abnormal history and physical exam findings

  e) Assessment of problems (dx, ddx, A, R/O, etc.)

  f) Doctor's treatment plan

  g) Client's acceptance, waiver or deferral of each element

  h) Diagnostics conducted with results

  i) Medication/prescriptions (with full SIG)

  j) Return/recheck/reminder/recall expectations

The above information could be streamlined, but liability would increase with deletion of critical information. The goal is not to enter the least data possible but rather to pursue prompts and formats which minimize keystroke requirements for entering the essential medical information.

A main system should include:

a) Presenting signs (client concerns)

b) New or existing client

c) New or existing patient (plus other pet screens for the household)

d) New or existing sign/concern

e) Ancillary wellness needs (vaccines, heartworm, FeLV, etc.)*

f) History

g) Examination (± diagnostic testing)*

h) Case assessment (What are we going to treat for?)

i) Supplemental testing needs*

j) Medications (full medical directions)* and treatments*

k) Dispensing*/prescribing action (full medical directions)

l) Client education

m) Next visit expectations (telephone and mail expectations too)

* Denotes a potential invoicing linkage requirement.

Hierarchy of data as proposed by most computer vendors skips "a" through "g" above. Veterinarians who want to retain their active licensure in practice cannot skip these steps. Line "h" may be the master problem, or might be a commitment to treat symptomatically if the client waived the diagnostic plan. Flexibility will be critical at this juncture.

- Computer templates for physical exams are not realistic. They can be too limited in some areas (e.g., some systems restrict respiratory system to lungs) and too broad in others (some systems call for a mucous membrane evaluation for every organ system).

I am not picking on any one computer system, but you need something a bit more innovative and creative than what we have been provided. If you want to attract the quality clients to your "new system," stay on paper until the computer database becomes relational.

Chapter 6:
How to Work with
Banks and Credit Bureaus

What bankers want to know about you

by Ross D. Clark, DVM, and Will Novak, DVM, MBA, a practice management consultant with Veterinary Management Concepts

Getting a loan from today's banks can be difficult, especially with the banking industry recovering from the wounds of the 1980s. Past events have made lending institutions re-evaluate the risks of loans; thus, they require more information about your financial position than ever before. The factors important to your banker demand serious investigation. Don't let a balance sheet technically derail your next loan application.

In the past, bank loan decisions were light-years more subjective than they are today. Here is a prime example: In the summer of 1960, when I (Ross Clark) was a second-year student at KSU College of Veterinary Medicine, I had an intense desire to purchase a red 1958 Chevrolet Impala convertible with a continental kit on the back. This car belonged to the Chevrolet dealer's wife in my home town, and it had only 14,000 miles on the odometer.

The asking price was $1,400. I had three jobs for the summer: night watchman for Farm Bureau, morning construction worker and afternoon necropsy room assistant. I felt I could sell my 1955 Ford for $500 and easily pay the $900 balance. I approached one banker on the north side of Poyntz Avenue in Manhattan, Kansas; and he told me my plan was silly. I should not even consider such a purchase with three more years of college left. He asked, "What would happen if you became ill?" Driven by intense desire, I walked directly across the street to another bank and talked to a younger loan officer, who, incidentally, knew my anatomy professor. He phoned the professor. Thirty minutes later, I had my loan.

Even today, it's not a good idea to give up after talking to only one banker. Bankers have become more objective than they were in the '60s, '70s and '80s but there is still a certain amount of subjectivity in their lending. If you know in your heart that your project is sound, your commitment will be evident and a good banker will eventually make your loan. Don't give up until you have talked to at least five banks. Ask each banker to explain specifically why a loan was turned down. Then use what you learn to improve your next presentation.

According to my co-author, Dr. Will Novak, each lending institution has its own specific criteria for determining the importance to be placed on each portion of a financial statement; however, similar categories and computer formulas for evaluating loan risk have emerged. These factors have been combined to create a financial model that can be rated on a scoring system.

The six main areas considered by the model are:

1. Cash flow

2. Collateral

3. Liquidity

4. Debt to worth ratio

5. Trends of the practice

6. Management

The scoring system in this specific model rates the risk of a loan from 0 to 60 points, with a minimum of 35 points required for a loan approval. This system is used by approximately 50 to 60 percent of national banks, primarily those on the East and West Coasts. Independents and smaller national banks use their own internal risk rating systems, which are set by underwriting guidelines from their corresponding regulatory agencies. All contemporary bankers are moving away from collateral-based loans to cash-flow- and ratio-based loans.

Bankers have become more objective then they were in the '60s, '70s and '80s but there is still a certain amount of subjectivity in their lending.

All ratios in this model are compared with Robert Morris and Associates (RMA) annual statement studies. RMA is the most widely utilized book of financial comparisons available to banks. It can be obtained by writing Robert Morris and Associates at One Liberty Place, Suite 2300, Philadelphia, PA 19103-7398; or by calling 215-851-9100.

1. Cash flow

Cash flow has a maximum allowable point value of 15 in this model and is made up of two ratio calculations:

Earnings before interest and taxes (EBIT)/interest expense:
This ratio measures the clinic's ability to meet interest payments.
For example, a practice with earnings of $100,000 (after a fair salary
and fair rent are subtracted) and interest payments of $20,000
would have a ratio of 6.0 ($120,000/$20,000). RMA cites 1.6 to 9.2
with a mean of 4.1 as normal. A ratio of 5.0 would be acceptable.

Cash flow/current maturity: This ratio measures the cash
available from the business (including noncash aspects of depreciation and amortization) to cover current long-term debt. It is a
good indicator of additional debt capacity. For example, a practice with earnings of $100,000 plus depreciation of $10,000 and
amortization of $10,000 and a current portion of long-term debt of
$30,000 would have a ratio of 4.0 ($120,000/$30,000). RMA recom-
mends a range of 1.3 to 4.4, so a ratio of 4.0 would be very good.

2. Collateral

Collateral carries up to 12 points and is based on the appraised
or estimated market value multiplied by a percentage. The percentage used will range from 50 percent to 80 percent, depending
on the type of asset.

Assets include cash, equipment, inventory and accounts receivable. Most veterinary clinics tend to be low in collateral because
a large portion of their total value lies in goodwill. Be sure your
accountant and your banker are made aware of the market value
rather than book value in this area. They tend to use book value
because it is the only information available, since market value is
not a component of a typical balance sheet. As your practice
matures, however, book value has less relationship to the true
value of your assets, because some assets such as stainless steel
cages, surgery tables and multipurpose tubs actually appreciate
in value. Also, many items such as stainless steel screws and
plates and other surgery supplies have been expensed and aren't
depreciated or carried on the inventory. Market value can be

determined by independent equipment appraisers, based on current replacement costs adjusted for age and wear. Include equipment lists with market value in your business plan, and update these as necessary.

3. Liquidity

Liquidity is determined by four different ratios and carries a maximum of 11 points. The ratios included are the current ratio, the quick ratio, the sales/accounts receivable ratio and the sales/net working capital ratio.

The *current ratio* divides total current assets by total current liabilities. A clinic with cash of $5,000, accounts receivable of $45,000 and inventory of $10,000 would have assets of $60,000. If current liabilities are $30,000, then the ratio would be 2.0. Because accounts receivable are included, a clinic with high accounts receivable will have a higher ratio. RMA found ratios of 0.6 to 4.8 (median = 1.2) for practices grossing less than $1 million, and 1.3 to 3.6 (median = 2.1) for practices grossing more than $1 million. A ratio of 2.0 would be acceptable.

The *quick ratio* adds the cash and accounts receivable and divides the total by the total current liabilities. The quick ratio is considered a more conservative estimate of liquidity. A clinic with accounts receivable of $25,000, cash of $5,000 and current liabilities of $30,000 would have a quick ratio of 1.0 ($30,000/$30,000). The RMA survey found quick ratios of 0.3 to 3.0 (median = 0.8) in practices grossing up to $1 million in sales, and 0.8 to 2.2 in practices grossing more than $1 million. In this example, a ratio of 1.0 would receive a good rating.

The *sales/accounts receivable (AR) ratio* determines the number of times your accounts receivable turn over during the year. The higher the turnover, the shorter the time between sales and cash collection. A clinic with an AR of $25,000 and a gross of $400,000 will have an AR ratio of 16.0. RMA lists ratios of 31.9 to 240.5 for practices grossing under $1 million, and 27.2 to 79.5 for practices grossing over $1 million. A turnover of 16 times per year would be considered poor.

The *sales/net working capital ratio* indicates whether a clinic is over-trading or, conversely, carrying more liquid assets than needed. The goal is to be near the mean and not at one end of the scale or the other. A clinic grossing $400,000 with a working capital of $40,000 (AR $25,000 + cash $5,000 + inventory $10,000 minus (-) current liabilities $30,000) would have a ratio of 40.0 ($400,000 / $10,000). RMA lists ratios of 12.9 to (-) 43.1 (mean = 95.5) for practices under $1 million, and 11.3 to 767.8 (mean = 35.6) for practices over $1 million. A sales/net working capital ratio of 40.0 would be good.

4. Debt to worth ratio

The d*ebt/worth ratio* carries a weight of 10 points. It is calculated by dividing the total liabilities by tangible net worth. This ratio expresses the relationship between capital contributed by the creditors and that contributed by the clinic owner.

The desire of any lending institution is to have an applicant with a low debt/worth ratio. A practice with total liabilities of $90,000 and tangible worth of $90,000 ($25,000 AR, $5000 cash, $50,000 equipment and $10,000 inventory) would have a ratio of 1.0. RMA found ratios of 0.9 to 25.4 (mean = 3.5) in practices grossing less than $1 million, and ratios of 0.4 to 2.0 (mean = 1.2) in practices grossing over $1 million. A ratio of 1.0 would receive good marks.

5. Trends

It is very important for the borrower to provide a strong explanation of trends and anticipated changes, including what the trends are and why they are occurring. This is very important to a banker. Discuss these trends in one section of your business plan. The trends analysis carries a value of eight points and is calculated by percentage changes in these four ratios: current ratio, debt/ worth ratio, EBIT/interest expense ratio and cash flow/sales ratio. Changes in these ratios indicate an improving or declining situation.

6. Management

The management area carries a total of four points and is a subjective value based on the experience and background of the owner. This value will vary with veterinarians, depending on length of time in practice, other business education and experience. Large practices can gain points if they have management staff members with CPA or MBA degrees.

Final score:

The subtotals from each area are added to get a final score. A final score of 50 to 60 points (See commercial credit scoring sheet on page 236) is considered excellent and practically ensures loan approval; whereas, a final score of 35 points or less practically ensures loan denial. This model would appear to make each and every loan approval an exacting science, but some flexibility still exists. Most models permit adjustments and some bankers consider factors that aren't included in the following model.

Commercial Credit Scoring Sheet
Veterinary Management Concepts

Cash Flow	Amt. 19X1	Amt. 19X2	RMA Value	Assgn.Pts.	Max Pts.
EBIT/Int. Exp.	7.00	9.00	1.6-9.2	7	
Cashflow/Cur.Mat	3.17	4.00	1.3-4.4	8	
				15	15
Collateral	$71,250.00	$71,250.00		8	12
Liquidity					
Current	1.08	1.33	0.6-4.8	2	
Sales-A/R	20.00	17.5	31.9-240.5	0	
Sales/NWC	120.00	35.00	−43.1-12.9	0	
Quick	0.067	0.083	0.3-3.0	2	
				4	11
Debt/Worth					
Debt/Worth	0.89	0.80	0.9-25.4	6	10
Trends					
Current	1.08	1.33	0.6-4.8	2	
Debt/Worth	0.89	0.80	0.9-25.4	0	
EBIT/Int. Exp.	7.00	9.00	1.6-9.2	2	
Cash flow/Sales	3.17	4.00	1.3-4.4	2	
				6	8
Management: DVM owner				2	4

Summary:	Assgn. Pts.	Max Pts.
Cash Flow	15	15
Collateral	8	12
Liquidity	4	11
Debt to Worth	6	10
Trends	6	8
Management	2	4
Total	41	60

Excellent	54-60
Above Average	45-53
Average	33-44
Watch	21-32
Substandard	10-20
Doubtful	0-9

Cash	$ 5,000.00	$ 5,000.00
Earnings	75,000.00	100,000.00
Interest Payments	12,500.00	12,500.00
Depreciation	10,000.00	10,000.00
Amortization	10,000.00	10,000.00
Current Long-term Debt	30,000.00	30,000.00
Long-term Debt	30,000.00	30,000.00
Fixed Assets	95,000.00	95.000.00
Current Liabilities	300,000.00	350,000.00
Gross Sales	30,000.00	30,000.00
Accounts Receivable	15,000.00	20,000.00
Inventory	12,500.00	15,000.00
Owner desires loan of $100,000 for expansion		

Key concepts and precautions

As you can see, ratios highlight items that may or may not be on a traditional balance sheet. If you are on a cash basis, accounts receivable may not be included on your balance sheet; thus, your banker may erroneously assume that you have no accounts receivable. Accounts receivable are an important component of working capital and many of the asset values are used in these ratio calculations. Cash on hand is also a very important component of total assets and working capital. Most veterinarians take all the cash out of their practices for personal debt service or for personal savings. Be careful to include retirement funds in your assets if they belong to the partnership or corporation.

Encourage your banker to use or be aware of current market value of equipment rather than its book value. A stainless steel surgery table that may have cost $375 twenty years ago would now cost $1,400. The book value is probably $0. Be sure to include an assets list at market value when you ask your banker if he or she can use market value. Bankers just want to get paid, so include a footnote about cross purchase life insurance available in case of death.

Veterinarians also tend to have hidden assets in stainless steel plates, screws and hand tools that were expensed rather than depreciated or inventoried. Again, tangible assets are a key component of the ratios your banker will be using. A $10,000 asset oversight could easily throw a ratio from above average to below average and from acceptable to unacceptable as a loan risk. Before you visit your banker for a loan application, know how your ratios stack up against national averages, and be prepared to explain ratios that don't measure up. You might need to point out that some of the RMA ratios are based on the values of only a few practices.

As the number-crunching abilities of computers grow, we believe that the entire field of veterinary practice management will become more objective and numbers-driven. Most certainly, so will loan applications and loan approvals. Don't let your dreams get sidetracked by misunderstood or miscalculated ratios. Better yet, knock your banker's socks off by presenting him with the financial data that really matters!

Source:

Clark, Kathy. Vice President Commercial Loans. First Bank Systems, Fargo, North Dakota. Personal Communication with Dr. Clark. Fall 1994.

What you need to know about bankers

by Ross D. Clark, DVM

As a practicing veterinarian, you may be overlooking some free business advice. Bankers deal with so many businesses that they've learned which business practices work and which don't. Recent changes in the financial world have given banks a renewed interest in serving professionals. Bankers call this new interest in small businesses "personal banking" or "relationship banking," but the intent is always to develop client confidence in an individual banker. You can build on this relationship, which can lead to increased practice profitability.

Four important concepts to keep in mind:

1. Do your homework.
2. Pick your banker; don't let your banker pick you.
3. Understand the basics of lending.
4. Know what your banker expects from you.

Choosing your banker

Bankers should be selected with care. The best way to choose one is to interview him or her for the job.

Start your discussion with a brief review of your background; good bankers want to know about you and your interests. Ask candidates to tour your office. If he or she refuses, find another banker. While you're conducting the tour, candidates can evaluate the intangibles that don't appear in a financial statement (e.g., neat, clean, professional facility; competent, courteous staff). Point out that stainless steel tubs, surgery tables and cages appreciate in value rather than depreciate.

The most important thing you can get from your prospective banker is his or her commitment to assume personal responsibility for your banking relationship. Although your banker can't personally handle all of your transactions, he or she can assume personal responsibility for identifying and resolving your account problems.

Your banker should provide names of others you can contact when he or she is unavailable; there should always be someone charged with looking out for you.

Will your banker watch out for your interests as you use other services—tax payments, loan payments and deposits? Every bank produces a series of exception reports highlighting potential customer problems, ranging from overdrawn accounts to non-posted deposits. Will your banker review these reports and initiate action that protects your interests? If your checking account is overdrawn, will he or she work with you to identify the cause before checks are returned?

You can ask your banker for help in just about any area of your business. Ask your banker for recommendations for lawyers, accountants and builders. Ask for a list of builders who are still on good terms with their clients after building completion. Your banker's recommendations reflect the integrity and financial strength of the business people with whom he or she has worked closely.

Ask for a description of deposit services. You'll quickly find that most banks offer nearly identical services, although each will offer certain twists to their products.

What your banker expects from you

As a financial professional, your banker expects to be treated with respect. Your banker also expects a relationship based upon honesty, directness and shared interest in the success of your practice. After you've chosen a banker, respect his or her time. Make it clear that you'll call him or her only for important matters and will call his or her assistants to resolve minor problems. Don't argue over incidental service charges; most of them are customary. If you think that incidental fees are getting too high or too frequent, make an appointment to review your account and to discuss how charges can be reduced or eliminated.

Writing a winning business plan

"It's no longer what 'shoulda been' or what 'oughta be' ... It's what's 'gotta be.'"

Bob Antin, CEO, Veterinary Centers of America

"If you fail to plan, you plan to fail."

Anonymous

According to a recent AT&T survey, 69 percent of the businesses surveyed agreed that a formal business plan is the major factor in helping to meet their business goals. Planning and replanning take a lot of work; and that's time you could spend paying the bills, talking to customers or handling employee issues. That's not laziness; it's the reality of trying to run a business. Yet 60 percent of companies reporting growth in the past two years said they "used formal business plans in their daily operations."

Starting your own practice can be the most scary, courageous, satisfying and rewarding step of your career. But realizing the American dream requires lots of hard work, not to mention determination, tenacity, enthusiasm, flexibility, imagination and responsibility.

Opening your own practice also requires a business plan, which may, in fact, be the most important document of your business career. It takes time, effort and money to prepare such a plan; but it can mean the difference between success and failure.

Take this to the bank

A complete and detailed business plan, accompanied by a loan proposal, can be a powerful money-raising tool. Your plan should include the following:

- A summary of your professional career.

- A description of your business philosophy and how you plan to manage your practice.

- A demographic study, as well as an evaluation of your clinic's chances for success in a given location.

- A traffic study of your site. In the past, we assumed the more traffic, the better; but that's not always true anymore. The heaviest, fastest traffic may be on its way out of town. That works fine for a fast-food place; but a veterinary clinic needs slower, local traffic. Potential clients should see you on their local, everyday routes, and be able to turn into your location without fear of a rear-end collision during rush-hour traffic.

Your finished business plan must be well organized, easy to read, factual and logical. It should run 25 to 30 double-spaced typewritten pages, with adequate appendices for illustration and detail. Such a plan lets prospective capital sources know that you've given deep and serious consideration to your business potential and that you're organized in your internal affairs.

A demographic primer

To illustrate the value and importance of demographic studies, let's take a look at a typical location that my company, Veterinary Management Concepts, would analyze and the types of information we would look at.

1. *Income data*: The first step in our analysis is to look at the total income generated in the study site. Ideally, the gross community income of an area should average $80 million per veterinarian. Of course, you can practice in an area with a lower figure, but you'll probably run into fairly intense competition.

In our sample site, the 1987 census shows two full-time equivalent veterinarians within a 10-mile radius. Our research indicates 20,630 households and a median family income of $29,826. The gross income of the area is therefore $615,310,380 (20,630 x $29,826). If another veterinarian were to move into the area, the gross community income would become $205,103,460 per veterinarian ($615,310,380 ÷ 3).

These calculations show that this site has great potential and will support an above-average practice. In fact, this area could support several more veterinarians. We rarely find such a wonderful site. If we do find such a site, we know that a veterinary hospital in this location is practically assured success.

2. *Pet-ownership data*: The second step of the analysis is based on the number of pet-owning households in the area. To prepare these calculations, you should assume that:

- 50 percent of the households own either a dog or a cat.
- The average number of pets per pet-owning household is 1.6.
- 60 to 75 percent of pet owners will take their pets in for veterinary services.
- The potential amount spent in a full-service hospital is $120 per pet per year. Full service includes boarding, grooming, pet food sales and 24-hour emergency service. The national average for veterinarians not offering full service is $78 per pet per year.

To determine the site potential, follow this formula:

[(number of households ÷ 2) x 1.6 pets x 0.75 x $100)] ÷ number of veterinarians = average gross income per practitioner.

Applying this formula to our sample area with 20,630 households and three veterinarians, you'll find an average gross income of $495,120 per veterinarian. ([(20,630 ÷ 2) x 1.6 x 0.75 x $120)] ÷ 3). The national average gross income per small-animal veterinarian per year is $169,999.

Clearly, the site we've explored has excellent potential. The numbers in your area will differ, but your business plan will work harder for you if you research and document what's possible in the site you've chosen.

Making the decision to open your own practice is never easy, even if you've done everything possible to ensure your success. I took courage in the wisdom of Theodore Roosevelt when I quit my job in Phoenix and moved to Tulsa to open my own practice in 1966.

Roosevelt, speaking to the Hamilton Club in 1899, said:

> "Far better it is to dare mighty things, to win glorious triumphs, even though checkered by failure, than to rank with those poor spirits who neither enjoy much, nor suffer much, because they live in the great twilight that knows not victory nor defeat."

Beef it up with a market survey

How can you determine if the site you've chosen will draw enough clients for a successful practice? The place to start is a study of the demographics of the area. You should be able to track down these figures through marketing analysis firms, real estate offices, the chamber of commerce or your local library. One such firm that we use is CACI at 1815 N. Ft. Myer Dr., Arlington, VA 22209. Their telephone number is 1-800-292-2224.

Current market projections for a veterinary clinic usually assume a five-mile radius as the area where the majority of your business will originate. However, in the example shown below, which is based on an actual site, I used a 10-mile radius

because of the area's low population density. The following
chart reflects the demographic details that will be most useful
in your business plan.

10-mile radius	1989 Census	1993 Census
Population	56,232	57,375
Households	20,630	22,222
Median family income	$29,826	$35,389
Average age	34.9	35.3
Household Income Levels		
$ 0-9,999	20.3%	17.2%
$10,000-14,999	10.1%	8.6%
$15,000-24,999	17.5%	16.0%
$25,000-34,999	18.7%	14.4%
$35,000-49,999	19.9%	20.7%
$50,000-74,999	10.2%	14.7%
$75,000 and up	3.4%	8.3%

On the expense side

You can build a convincing business plan for your proposed
practice using demographic information, but the bank will also be
interested in your expenses. To give you an idea of what kind of
information you'll need, the chart on page 246 projects expenses
for a solo practice expected to gross $120,000 the first year.

Property rent will be too high at the beginning; however, it will
fall in line when practice gross doubles to $240,000 annually.
Then rent will be 8.25 percent of gross, which is acceptable.
Provide all assumptions in written form attached to the pro
forma—any evidence of revenues and expenses (e.g., lease agreements, etc.) is appreciated.

Income Statement: Services—$120,000 gross income

Expenses	Monthly	Yearly	% of gross
Property rental	$1,750	$21,000	17.50 %
Utilities (average)	900	10,800	9.00
Telephone:			
yellow pages	150	1,800	1.50
basic service (3 lines)	160	1,920	1.60
long distance	50	600	0.50
answering service	58	696	0.58
paging service	11	132	0.11
Maintenance	150	1,800	1.50
Grounds keeping	50	600	0.50
Other	100	1,200	1.00
Rubbish	25	300	0.25
Computer supplies	50	600	0.50
Printing (invoices, cards, etc.)	35	420	0.35
Office supplies	167	2,004	1.67
Postage	21	252	0.21
CPA	21	252	0.21
Drugs and professional supplies	917	11,004	9.17
Lab expenses	125	1,500	1.25
Pet food	25	300	0.25
Uniforms	10	120	0.10
Cleaning/laundry	4	48	0.04
Licenses	3	36	0.03
Dues	8	96	0.08
Subscriptions	7	84	0.07
Rabies tags	4	48	0.04
Continuing education	8	96	0.08
Medical reimbursement	250	3,000	2.50
Property insurance	58	696	0.58
Professional insurance	10	120	0.10
Staff Wages			
($5/hr, 173 hrs/mo., 3 employees)	2,595	31,140	25.95
FICA	56	672	0.56
Benefits	75	900	0.75
Total	$ 7,853	$ 94,236	78.53 %
Owner's professional salary	$ 2,000	$ 24,000	20.00 %
Total expenses	$ 9,853	$118,236	
Net to owner	$ 147	$ 1,764	1.47 %

Source:

Anderson, R. *Veterinary Economics.* Expense Survey. November
    1994: 23.

What *not* to do in a business plan

by J. Tol Broome, Jr.

A few cautionary tips from a commercial loan officer:

- Don't submit a rough copy. A coffee-stained business plan or one with words crossed out tells the prospective lender or investor that you don't take your proposal seriously.

- Don't use stale information. Outdated financial information or industry comparisons raise doubts about your planning ability.

- Don't make unsubstantiated assumptions. Be prepared to explain the "whys" of every point in your plan.

- Don't paint too much blue sky. Failing to consider prospective pitfalls can make your ideas look unrealistic. List potential risks to repayment—provide mitigators to those risks.

- Don't ignore the financial information. Even if an outside source prepares the projections, you must fully understand and be prepared to discuss all of the information in the plan.

- Don't forget outside influences. When you make your request, be prepared to discuss the potential impact of competitive factors as well as the economic environment.

- Don't assume you won't have to stake your own money. The investor or lender will likely expect you to have some equity capital invested in your business.

- Don't be unwilling to guarantee loans personally. If you won't stand behind your practice, why should the bank?

- Don't introduce the plan with a demand for unrealistic funding terms. The lender wants to know about the viability of the practice before discussing the terms of the funding request.

- Don't focus on collateral over projected earnings. Even for a cash-secured loan, the banker looks toward projected profits for loan repayment—that's why it's important to emphasize cash flow.

This article has been excerpted from "Business plans: plotting your road map to success" which appeared in the July 1994 issue of *Veterinary Economics*.

Protecting your credit rating

by Jan Coody, MBA, Hospital Administrator at Woodland PetCare Centers

Having a good credit rating is very important to veterinarians. When applying for a loan, a credit card, a mortgage, renting a car or just sending flowers, your credit history is going to be checked. It could make the difference in your ability to expand or even continue in your practice.

Almost all adults are on the records of three main credit reporting companies: TRW, TransUnion and Equifax. These credit bureaus have little government regulation, are known to make many errors and be quite unfair. They can contain very personal information that is available to the public. Nearly anyone who wants a report on you can get it. Do not let erroneous or misleading credit reports ruin your credit. Know your credit rating.

Your credit history is so important, even if you have good credit you should periodically check your credit report. Getting your report can sometimes be difficult. Only recently have the credit bureaus acknowledged in their policies that credit reports are available to the person they are reporting on. Remember, as sole proprietors and partners in our practices, leases and bank loans are often listed on our personal or individual social security number. We know of very large hospitals where leases and bank loans for the partnership are still listed on the partner's credit report. Even when you have no late payments, too many credit cards and accounts can hurt your credit rating. Potential credit grantors may weigh monthly debt service against your personal income, not your practice income.

Getting your credit report

There are two versions of your credit report. One is the consumer report that you get when checking your credit yourself and the other is a professional version that a lender receives when checking your credit.

Your personal credit file should be free for review but often they are not. You need to check on the amount of the fee. If you have recently been rejected for a loan there is a law stating that you are entitled to a free copy of the report used to deny you credit within the last 30 days.

When writing for your credit report make three copies of your request, one for each of the major companies. Each company maintains separate files that can contain different information. It is important to include your Social Security number. You will need to verify your identity by enclosing a copy of your utility bill, credit card bill or driver's license with your current address.

If the information you have has an old address on it be sure and identify it as a former address. Also be sure to sign and date your letter. If your name has changed make a note to the credit bureau of the change. Send your letters to the following credit bureaus:

Equifax Information Service
Customer Correspondence
P.O. Box 740193
Atlanta, GA 30374-0193
(800) 685-1111

TRW
P.O. Box 749-029
Dallas, TX 75374
(800) 392-1122

TransUnion
P.O. Box 8070
North Olmsted, OH 44070-8070
(800) 922-5490

You should make a copy of all of your correspondence and use certified/return receipt mail. You might want to keep a log of the date you sent your requests so you can follow up if needed.

If you do not get a response within a month, make an extra copy of the letter you sent and send it along with a cover letter stating you have not gotten a response in over a month to:

Federal Trade Commission (FTC)
Credit Bureau Complaints
Pennsylvania Ave. and 6th St. N.W.
Washington, DC 20580

You should also send a copy of this letter to the FTC to the credit bureau.

At the present time, TRW will send a free credit report once a year, but TransUnion and Equifax charge for their reports. Check with TransUnion or Equifax as to what their fees are and enclose a money order to cover them. A money order is better than a check as there will not be an additional waiting period for the check to clear the bank.

If you are writing to a credit bureau because you were turned down for credit or insurance, include this in your letter. The institution that turned you down is required to tell you which credit bureau issued the report although they are not required to give you a copy. This report will be free from all three of the credit bureaus. Let them know what you were rejected for, the name of the rejector and the date of rejection. Be sure to make this request within 30 days of the rejection, although TRW has extended the time limit to 60 days.

The credit report you will receive on yourself is often different as it is not as detailed as the reports sent to lending professionals. These reports sent to the professionals are called "infiles." Some derogatory information, such as the timing of late payments, is difficult to read or omitted on TRW and Equifax consumer reports. TRW gives a national risk score of your credit worthiness between 0 to 1,000, with 0 being the best credit. This number is left off of consumer reports. TransUnion gives the same report to the consumer and the professionals. Companies that subscribe to credit bureaus or their subsidiaries have agreements not to give consumers a copy of their own "infiles."

There are laws that a person's credit is only to be accessed by those contemplating a business transaction who are thereby in need of this information. It is simple, however, for a detective, landlord or employer to get your "infiles" by supplying your name and Social Security number.

If you need your files faster, they will fax it the same day it is ordered. A quick way to get your "infiles" is to register as a prospective employer or landlord with the local credit bureau. You may be able to register the same day you call by using the fax machine. Once you are registered, you can have credit reports sent by fax or mail within hours.

The cost of these services range in price from $2.75 to $15. There are companies that will order them for you at a substantial markup, charging as much as $50. These local credit bureaus are listed in your yellow pages under credit, or you might ask a mortgage or other lending professional which company he or she uses.

The credit report that mortgage companies use is called a full factual report and it combines two "infiles." TRW and TransUnion are the two most commonly used reporting agencies, although some companies use all three of the credit bureaus. The full factual report often costs around $50 and a credit bureau employee makes calls to the employer, landlord, present mortgage company and others about items on the report that seem to merit verification.

If you have items on your report that you are disputing, it is best to deal with the credit bureau directly and not list them on your mortgage application.

Reading the credit report

Credit reports come in many different styles but they are all derived from the three main credit bureaus. Each of the three have different formats as do the regional credit bureaus, which resell from the three major ones.

The flip side of the report has information that helps you understand the report. The credit bureaus also publish information to help you read their reports. Understandably the information they prepare tends to de-emphasize harmful information which discourages challenges to the reporting system by suggesting ineffective dispute resolution methods.

TRW

The consumer credit report has some but not all of the derogatory items identified with an asterisk to the left of the creditor's name and in the right-hand "Status/Payments" column. The disadvantage is that the consumer report leaves out valuable information that is on the professional report.

The TRW Updated Credit Profile Disclosure is what you will get in response to a written dispute of bad credit items. It usually only lists the items that are in dispute.

The left-hand side of the credit profile has three columns: Pos, Non, Neg. Each credit item is assigned to one column and has a letter that refers to how it was verified. If it is Pos (positive), the credit is good. If it is Neg (negative), it is hurting your credit rating. If it is Non, it is likely to be bad. This designation is usually applied to items that were at some point late or delinquent but are now up-to-date or paid. Several of these "Non" rated marks could disqualify you from getting a mortgage or business loan.

The name of the creditor is found to the right of the Pos, Non and Neg columns. The account number is in a column on the right side. This number is important for communication with the creditor or credit bureaus.

The account status is found under the creditor's name. This line gives the details of the Pos, Non and Neg ratings. Terms used for good credit are CURR ACCT, meaning a good and open account. PAID ACCT is a closed good account that is now paid. The PAID SATIS is also a closed good account. Almost any other rating is undesirable to have on your report. Look closely at any credit settlement that does not change the account status to one of these three.

Current accounts that result in a Non rating even though the account is up-to-date can be harmful to your credit rating. CUR WAS 30 is an account that is presently on time but was 30 days late at least once in the last seven years. Other designations of additional days late are CUR WAS 60, 90, 120, 150, 180. A designation of CUR WAS 30-2 means that the account was 30 days late at least two times. CUR WAS COL is a current account that was in collection at some point in the past seven years. CUR WAS DL is a current account that was delinquent.

Delinquent means that collection efforts were made. CUR WAS FOR is a current account that was in foreclosure. CR LN CLOS is an account that has been closed. These closures are often requested by consumers, but no matter who requests the account be closed, this status often includes the additional phrase "subscriber request," which means that the creditor requested it to be closed.

All delinquent accounts will have a Neg rating. These are designated by DELIQ 60 meaning the account is now 60 days delinquent. Other variations of additional days late include DELIQ 90, 120, 150, 180. DEL WAS 90 means the account was 90 days delinquent and is now 60 days delinquent. DEL WAS 120 is an account that was 120 days delinquent and is now 90, 60 or 30 days delinquent. GOV CLAIM is a claim for the insured part of a defaulted student loan. CHARGE OFF is an account that is written off as a loss for tax purposes by the creditor.

The amount owed on a delinquent account can be an extremely low amount of money but can be severely damaging to your credit. PD CHARGE OFF is a charge-off that you have paid. Even though it has been paid this credit status is still very derogatory.

The status date refers to the last reporting to the credit bureau on the item. If the date is within the last three months it means that the creditor keeps your account in the current files. If the status date is over a year old the creditor has probably put your account in the archives. These accounts are less likely to be verified when challenged.

A TRW "infile" has some differences to look for from the consumer credit report or the updated credit profile. There are no misleading Pos, Non or Neg ratings. All harmful credit items are marked with an asterisk in the far left-hand column. The account number is below the creditor name and under that is the subscriber number. Sometimes the account number is truncated (some numbers dropped off) to limit fraud. The account status is found at the far-right of the page. The terms are the same as on the credit profile but the "infile" lists the 24-month account history coded on two lines underneath the status terms.

An example:

CUR WAS 30-3
CCCCCCCCCCC1
11CCNNNCCCCC

The position of the letters and the numbers represents the last 24 months, with the upper left being the month of the status date being the most recent.

The "C" means a current account—that the payment was on time. The N means a current account with a zero balance—with no money owed. The "1" means the payment was 30 days late. On some reports, a "1" is used to represent an on-time payment which you can identify if the status term of an account with lots of "1s" reads current. If this rating is used, a "2" would refer to a payment that was 30 days late and a "3" would mean 90 days late.

There are several dates on the "infile." The status date is the important one and is located just to the left of the account status section on the most right column. This date indicates the last time that your file was updated to include account status terms. A status date of over a year indicates that an account is probably no longer active. The status date helps you interpret the 24-month history because it represents the top left account month on the 24-month section.

TransUnion

TransUnion's consumer reports and infiles to lending professionals are essentially the same. The creditor is found at the left margin. The number found just below the creditor's name—not the subscriber number just to the right of the creditor's name—is the account number. Account numbers, if credit cards, are truncated. At the far right of the page is the heading, type of account and MOP (method of payment). Account status rating is a letter: I, R, C or O followed by a number from 01 to 09. An "I" means installment credit, "R" means revolving credit, "C" means a line of credit on your checking account and "O" means an open account. An 09 rating is the worst credit and is usually reserved for charge-offs.

Anything but an 01 rating indicates bad credit. The second account status rating is a payment history—usually a two-line 24-month history and a historical status line of four numbers that summarize any late payments.

An example:

```
111111111121
11113211111
  48 2 1 0
```

The numbers represent the last 24 months, with the upper left being the most recent month. The number "1" means the payment was on time, the "2" means 30 days late, the "3" means 60 days late, the "4" means 90 days late and on up to "7" which is 180 days late. An X means no history report and a blank means no history is maintained. The historical status line of four numbers begins in the example with the number "48," which means the credit records go back 48 months. The next number represents the number of payments reported as 30 days late, which would be two in the example. The "1" represents how many payments were reported as 60 days late and the "0" is how many payments were reported as 90 days late. The historical status line can go back seven years.

The "date verified" column reveals how recently your credit was reported from the creditor. If the date verified is over a year old it probably means the account is inactive. The date verified also identifies the date of the top left month in the 24-month history so that you know what months are represented.

Equifax

The consumer report and infiles to lending professionals are essentially the same but have a slight variation in layout. The account number is in the second column from the left. The account status is found in the second column from the right side of the page. The status rating is designated by an I, O or R followed by a number from 1 to 9. An "I" means installment credit, "O" means open credit with relaxed payment terms and "R" means revolving credit. A "9" is the worst credit and usually means charge-offs. Anything but a "1" rating means bad credit.

Late payments are indicated underneath the creditor name by a line beginning >>> PRIOR PAYING HISTORY followed by a series of numbers and letters. If the account does not have this line there are no late payments.

An example:

>>>PRIOR PAYING HISTORY - 30(09)60(02)
90+(00)06/92-R2,04/92-R2,12/91-R3

The numbers in parentheses tell the number of times the account was 30 days, 60 days or more than 90 days late. In the example, the account was paid 30 days late a total of nine times,

60 days, two times and never 90 or more days late. The dates following those numbers show changes in the account status referring to when the delinquencies occurred. The worst status is the R3, which was given to the account when the two 60 days late were recorded in 12/91.

The right most column, "Date Reported," shows how recently the credit was reported from a particular creditor. If the date is more than a year old, an inactive account is probably indicated. Again, credit bureaus report bad credit for many years, usually seven.

Repairing your credit report

Credit repair can be done by disputing derogatory items with the credit bureaus. The credit bureaus will often clear the record rather than spend the time necessary to go over an individual item. Often they will try to wear down your patience but you should be persistent and not give up.

Begin your dispute with a series of well-timed letters. You will have to dispute similar items on different credit reports as clearing an item on one credit bureau's records will not clear it on the other ones. But if you succeed in clearing an item off one report, you will more than likely succeed with the other credit bureaus. If you have three or fewer items to dispute with each bureau, then conduct the disputes concurrently.

Send your initial dispute letter. If you do not get a response within 30 days, send a second-notice letter. Ten days after the second-notice letter, send the FTC a dispute letter with a copy of the second-notice letter. Also send a copy of what you sent to the FTC to the credit bureaus.

When you get a response from the credit bureaus, if they have removed all the derogatory items that you disputed, your credit repair is done! If you are dealing with TRW, on the credit update it will state ABOVE ITEM DELETED or ITEM changed as above. This should read CURR ACC or PAID SAT or PAID ACC and not some lesser but still derogatory status. After responses from TransUnion or Equifax, check to see that the item is removed or else the 30-60-90 day late pay indicator will all read zero (0).

If some but not all of the derogatory items are removed, you will recognize on TRW's report a response of ITEM REMAINS, CONFIRMED BY SOURCE or the item is corrected to a lesser degree of lateness.

The response from TransUnion or Equifax if items are not repaired will remain unchanged, or be repeated without the 30-60-90 day indicators and the comment ITEM IN DISPUTE, or the item may have less severe 30-60-90 day indicators. Next you will need to send a second demand letter which specifically enumerates your consumer rights to dispute the uncorrected items.

The more specific complaints force the credit bureau to choose between an expensive investigation or clearing your credit. If none of the items are corrected, try not to be frustrated. This is a common delaying tactic. If TRW does this the update will state, ITEM REMAINS CONFIRMED BY SOURCE. TransUnion and Equifax will send new copies of your credit report with the disputed items unchanged.

If you have over three items to dispute you need to approach the process a little differently. Challenge items with the same procedures. But just take on two or three items at a time. You never want to dispute more than three items at a time with any one credit bureau.

It is best to dispute different items with different credit bureaus so that you can determine which will be removed most easily from your credit history. Then re-dispute the ones that are removed first with the other credit bureaus. Hold the items that did not come off to the side for re-disputing later.

If you have more items to dispute but there are only a few, you may want to re-dispute the original rejected items immediately and send a second dispute letter in which you will add the one or two new disputes to the original items that were not removed in the initial dispute. Credit bureaus are required by law to respond to all written disputes, but they are good at delaying tactics. If you are aware of them and can send the information they will request in the first place, it will save unnecessary delays for you.

They sometimes send a form letter asking you to prove identity by providing a utility bill or another form of identification. Include this in your first letter, making this request unnecessary. You might receive a form letter telling you they are investigating your complaint. Ignore this and proceed with the next letter. Another form letter they send could be to tell you the complaint is not specific enough. If your dispute is clear and legally sound, you should also ignore this and proceed.

Sometimes the credit bureau will just not answer. Be sure to use certified mail/return receipt. If you have not heard anything in six weeks, then start over by sending a copy of the letter but also send a copy to the FTC.

When sending your initial dispute letter, be sure to include your name, address, phone and Social Security number. Again, include a copy of a recent utility bill to prove who you are and that you are at your address.

In your opening paragraph state that there are errors, that these errors are hurting your credit and that these errors will cause you to suffer some specific loss. State what you personally stand to lose—an opportunity to purchase needed equipment for your practice, for instance.

Give the name of the creditor that reported the bad credit on you and your account number with that creditor. List each creditor, account number and dispute separately if you are disputing more than one. As stated earlier, do not dispute more than three items at a time.

You will want to give the reason the credit item is wrong. For example, you may have been confused with someone else. There may have been some sort of billing problem. Or you may be certain you always paid on time and have canceled checks. The credit bureaus will rarely correct an item if you accept blame and give a reason like being out of work or sick.

Sign your name to the letter and always remember to send the letter certified/return receipt.

After a month, if you have not had a response, make a copy of the first letter and the postal receipt from the certified letter, or at least note the date it was mailed. Start your next letter with a statement that this is the second time you are sending this request. Also send this letter certified/return receipt.

If after one month, you get no response, send a copy of the initial dispute letter, along with a copy of the green postal receipt. Add to the copy that this is the second time you are sending this. Again use certified/return receipt mail.

If you get a response from the credit bureau to your letters but they refuse to correct any of the items on the report, then you need to send another letter. The opening paragraph needs to convey that the complaints of errors in the credit report were ignored; the errors have hurt financially and are continuing to do so; and the ways in which you have been financially penalized for the error. State what you personally stand to lose because of the errors. Go into more detail as to the reason the item is wrong. Then explain that you are going to take stronger action if you do not get satisfaction, such as call your lawyer, or report the credit bureau to the FTC or your state attorney general.

If the credit bureau corrects some of the items but refuses to correct other items on your report, let them know that they corrected some items but not all. State that they were all wrong and that you understand that they are liable for errors. If they do not correct the mistake immediately you will take stronger action.

If the credit bureau corrects the errors you have sent to them and you want to add more at this time, your opening paragraph should thank them for correcting items, but state that you have found more errors that are hurting your credit. Again state that the errors will cause you a specific loss.

If you have not gotten any response from the credit bureaus after six weeks—which is the reasonable time period that the law gives them to respond—send a letter to the FTC informing them that the credit bureau will not respond to your complaint about errors in your credit report. Enclose a copy of your letter about the dispute and a copy of the certified/return receipt. Then send a copy to the credit bureau that is not responding. You may also want to send copies to your state attorney general's office or your state department of consumer affairs.

Some situations are best handled with the creditor who is reporting bad credit on you rather than going through the credit bureau. The advantages in going directly to the creditor are that the agreement to clear an item will clear it with all three credit bureaus at once; older items can be confirmed; and the grouped or scattered nature of the lateness in the 24-month history can be cleared. Grouped latenesses are sometimes attributed to one uncredited payment causing the next ones down the line to appear late.

In dealing with the creditor, do not make your arguments personal. Focus on the facts of the case and never get angry at the person you are dealing with. Let them know that you realize they are doing their job and they have responsibilities. Tell them the bad credit mark from their company is causing you some problem, such as not getting a mortgage. Ask for their help in the matter. State that you are a paying customer and plan to continue doing business with them. Let them know you are interested in resolving the credit problem and need their help. Offer some possible reasons why the item was not really late, or that there was a misunderstanding. They might be willing to offer a payment schedule in exchange for clearing the credit.

The Fair Credit Billing Act and the Fair Credit Reporting Act provide the rules for what is an on-time payment and what is a correct billing procedure. The existence of billing errors, which would mean you were not really late, will allow the creditor to ease the credit. Most companies will send you a letter to verify that they are correcting your credit and will notify the credit bureaus.

Many times negotiations with a creditor will help clear a negative credit item. A restrictively endorsed settlement is an agreement that acceptance of the check signifies that the account is paid in full or paid up-to-date and the derogatory items will be deleted with the major credit bureaus. A debt schedule settlement can help you negotiate by making regular payments to clear your credit as soon as you start paying the money back.

If your creditor negotiations are getting no response, you might want to consider a lawyer to get the settlement you need. When the attorney gets involved the creditor begins to worry about limiting liability. Many times they can negotiate an enforceable agreement that clears your credit in exchange for ending the dispute.

The need for a good credit status requires that you use vigilance to insure that your credit history is reported accurately. An understanding of credit reporting systems may prevent future financial problems and potential loss.

Source:

Bierman, T., and N. Wice. *The Guerrilla Guide to Credit Repair, How To Find Out What's Wrong With Your Credit Rating—And How To Fix It.* New York: St. Martin's Press, 1994.

Notes

Chapter 7:
Partnership and
Associate Agreements

Associate veterinarian contracts

by Ross D. Clark, DVM, and David Madden, JD, attorney in Overland Park, Kan.

The model contract found in the accompanying *Practice Workbook,* Section 3: Contracts, outlines a basic employee agreement. Associates and owners both will benefit from written agreements that clearly define duties, benefits, compensation, options and term of employment.

This is intended to be a model contract, and we recommend that you and your attorney use it as a reference for drafting your specific contracts. Many attorneys are not familiar with veterinary concerns, and because of this they end up spending too much of their time and our money drawing up contracts when they could be using more standard models.

Contracts are legally enforceable promises. There are basically two kinds of contracts: expressed and implied. An *expressed contract* is one where the terms are stated by the parties orally or in writing. An *implied contract* is one where the terms are derived from the contract of the parties.

The *requisites* of a contract are:

- Parties must be legally competent.

- There must be sufficient consideration.

- It must be performable.

- It must not be contrary to public policy.

The first requisite, *legal competence,* requires that the parties must be under no legal disability. For example, they must be of legal age and mentally competent.

Consideration means that some benefit must pass or accrue to all contracting parties such as money, the promise to do something or the promise to forbear from doing something.

A contract can be *performed* only if its objectives can be accomplished.

Contracts that are *contrary to the law or public policy* are either void or voidable and thus cannot be enforced legally.

The relationship between an employer and an employee is contractual. The contract of employment can be either expressed or implied. An employment contract between employer and employee is determined by the principles governing the formation of other contracts.

Whether the contract is oral or written, there must be mutual assent to the contract. It is often said that there must be a "meeting of the minds." The consent of the parties to the terms of an employment contract can be determined by circumstantial evidence. The performance of a contract by the parties is circumstantial evidence of the consent of the parties to the contract.

An *enforceable employment contract* must definitely state, orally or in writing, these three points:

- the parties to the contract;
- the kind of employment; and
- the compensation paid for employment.

The advantage of a written contract is that the terms can be enumerated clearly and concisely.

A written employment contract may be drawn up by one of three methods:

- The parties may draw a letter agreement, which is a broad-brush device and is usually not detailed.
- The parties may sign a "form" agreement. In this case, an employer draws a standard agreement for employees with the same duties and job classifications.
- The parties can draw a detailed contract that covers all conceivable points of employment. This method is usually tailored for individual employees, like new associates in veterinary hospitals.

The real importance of a contract is often never realized until you're standing before a judge who is interpreting its meaning.

Regardless of your contract method, be sure you don't plug square pegs into round holes. Each contract should be as individualized as time and money warrant. The real importance of a contract is often never realized until you're standing before a judge who is interpreting its meaning. If an agreement is important enough to write, you should consider its enforceability.

Every employment contract should:

- identify the parties;

- state the terms of the employment;

- describe the duties of the employee;

- detail the compensation to be paid to the employee, including salary and fringe benefits;

- state how and when the contract is terminated, such as by the death or disability of the employee; and

- include a covenant not to compete (optional).

Restrictive covenants

Initially, common law viewed restrictive covenants with disfavor and would not enforce them because they were seen as unfair restraints of trade. Today the courts, with some exceptions, have enforced reasonable covenants not to compete through injunctions.

Some state courts have said that when restrictive covenants are unreasonable in time, area or both, they fail completely and are not enforceable. Arizona, Arkansas, Georgia, Maine, Nebraska, South Carolina, Tennessee, Virginia and Wisconsin fall into this category. Five miles and five years have been considered reasonable in large cities for small-animal practices. Mixed- animal practice in a sparsely populated area may be restricted to 25 miles.

Other state courts may make an unreasonable covenant enforceable by striking its excessive language. This has occurred in Connecticut, Illinois, Indiana, New York, North Carolina, Pennsylvania, Rhode Island and West Virginia.

Puerto Rico and the states of Alaska, Colorado, Delaware, Florida, Hawaii, Idaho, Iowa, Kansas, Kentucky, Maryland, Massachusetts, Minnesota, Mississippi, Missouri, New Hampshire, New Mexico, New Jersey, Nevada, Ohio, Oregon, Texas, Utah, Vermont, Washington and Wyoming have enforced restrictive covenants when the enforcement was reasonable under the circumstances.

There are five states that prohibit restrictive covenants by statute: California, Montana, North Dakota, Oklahoma and South Dakota. In the case of these five states, you, an owner, may have other legal options to protect your practice and investment when hiring a new associate.

A less restrictive device is the "anti-solicitation covenant" which would prohibit the use of patient lists by departing employees.

Any contract, whether oral or written, should be fair to all parties to ensure its enforceability. It should accomplish the employer's purposes without oppressing the employee.

Associate compensation

by Ross D. Clark, DVM

In recent years, many practice owners and management consultants, myself included, have advocated paying associates a percentage of their individual gross production. The generally accepted total compensation package has consisted of 25 percent of the associate's gross, plus Workers' Compensation, FICA, health insurance, continuing education and vacation pay. Today, however, these numbers may be completely inappropriate for most practices.

Why? Because your ability to pay acceptable salaries is based on factors other than production. In fact, for an associate veterinarian working in an especially progressive practice with a state-of-the-art image, utilizing high ratios of lay/professional staff, a percentage as low as 12 percent may be a more viable alternative. On the other hand, for a veterinarian working in a new satellite shopping center practice with a part-time receptionist, no technician, no kennel assistants and very few clients, 30 percent of gross may not be enough professional pay.

What factors determine the best percentage for you? Before you assume that 25 percent is right for your practice, consider these six factors:

1. The total cost of your professional and lay staff

In setting compensation for the veterinarians in your practice, you face two challenges:

- determining a percentage of gross production figure that is fair to your associates; and

- making sure that your total employee costs (including a fair salary for yourself) don't exceed 40 percent of your hospital's entire production.

Lay staff percentage. Before you can decide on a fair percentage for your associate(s), you must first determine the percentage that goes to all lay staff. Assigning a figure to staff use is difficult because some associates use staff support much more extensively than others. In some hospitals, the costs for lay staff may run as high as 32 percent. To remain within the 40-percent guideline, management would be forced to pay an associate only eight percent of his or her gross.

This low associate percentage should raise a red flag: the staff may be overpaid or the hospital may have too many staff members. On the other hand, the staff may be so efficient that the associate doesn't have to handle as many duties; thus justifying a lower percentage for associate compensation.

Associate percentage. You should take into consideration how much staff support each associate requires. Smaller hospitals and solo-veterinarian clinics may find it easier to calculate the amount of staff support provided for each associate. In general, associates who work better alone should receive a higher percentage of the revenue they produce for the practice.

Benefits. For health insurance, I suggest paying $100 to $150 (1995 U.S. dollars) per month on each employee's policy. The employee should pay the balance of what he or she wants for coverage of spouse and children. Paying the same for each employee makes the company policy more equitable to unmarried employees. Disability and life insurance policies are not usually paid on behalf of associates.

I recommend that the clinic or hospital cover the registration fees for one state, one regional and one national meeting for each associate. But transportation, meals and lodging should be paid by the associate.

Total percentage. I have found that most practices hold total lay-staff costs at about 20 percent. The average practice holds total veterinary compensation, including benefits, at about 23 percent, putting total compensation about three percent over the 40-percent guideline. If your costs for lay staff run higher than 20 percent, be sure to consider all factors carefully before computing associate compensation based on production. One practice I know of showed a total personnel cost of 70 percent of gross last December—proof that personnel costs can get out of hand during slower times. Don't let your practice be surprised by winter!

2. The method you use to calculate production

A full-service hospital typically credits 75 percent of its total production to veterinarians and 25 percent to the hospital and lay staff (which includes boarding, pet food sales and some retail products). Grooming is labor-intensive, so remove any grooming expenses and revenue from this formula whenever possible. If you pay associates 50 percent or 100 percent of emergency calls, be sure to subtract that emergency call compensation from the associate's gross, or you will be paying more than 100 percent on those dollars.

To see how these production ratios can vary depending on the calculation method, look at the following examples. Each assumes a two-veterinarian hospital grossing $40,000 a month:

Hospital 1: The veterinarians in this hospital are credited with 90 percent of hospital gross, or $18,000 each. If their compensation package gives them 20 percent of gross production, each doctor will receive $3,600 a month plus benefits.

Hospital 2: The veterinarians in this hospital are credited with only 70 percent of the hospital's gross, or $14,000 each. If they receive 25 percent of gross, each will be paid $3,500 a month plus benefits.

As you can see, the methods used to calculate individual production can have a major impact on salary. In the case of Hospital 2, for example, 25 percent of gross is not better.

3. The amount of capital investment provided to boost associate production

Before you can establish any salary percentages, you must determine how much you've invested in your equipment and physical plant. For example, how much money must be earmarked for new equipment that will allow you to stay competitive in today's high-tech atmosphere?

As with a capital investment, a portion of each associate's gross production must be allocated to provide a fair return on your investment. Of course, you should determine a realistic return that doesn't penalize you as the investor or the clients who use the asset. Here again, giving your associate less than 25 percent of gross may be necessary. Why? Because with more sophisticated equipment and an upgraded physical plant, your associate will be more productive. The associate will be able to charge higher fees, so he or she will still make the same amount of money—or more. Remember, being able to perform more expensive procedures (e.g., ultrasonograms, computer-assisted electrocardiograms and IV pyelograms) not only leads to higher individual productivity; it improves the practice image.

4. The amount you've invested in marketing

You can have a new hospital, the best-trained staff and the finest equipment around; but if no one knows about you, you won't succeed.

You must conduct marketing programs that announce that your hospital offers the finest care, the newest equipment and the most qualified veterinarians. In these days of soaring costs, every dollar must count. Even the U.S. Postal Service's plans to raise the cost of a first-class letter can drastically affect your marketing efforts.

Your marketing budget should be large enough to accommodate contact with regular clients as well as new and potential clients. Without marketing, associate productivity may suffer; so be cautious when assigning compensation percentages.

5. The mix of services you provide

In general, a hospital that provides a wide range of services (e.g., grooming, obedience classes and in-house lab analyses) will have a higher staff labor cost as a percentage of gross. For instance, veterinarians usually are credited 100 percent for the lab work they order, whether the work is performed in-house (by veterinarian or staff) or by an outside lab. Of course, lab work performed by an outside lab will lower labor costs, but it won't result in increased net income to the practice owner. Veterinarians who work in hospitals that send a considerable amount of lab work to an outside lab should, therefore, receive a lower percentage of gross than those who perform most of their own lab analyses. Although performing the majority of lab work in-house may not raise practice revenue, this service may necessitate that you raise your total employee costs closer to or above 40 percent to account for the higher labor costs. (See Chapter 9: Managing miscellanies, "In-house lab equipment vs. professional lab services.")

Keep in mind, too, that while high-volume retail sales tend to lower overall labor costs as a percentage of gross, your costs of goods increase.

6. Non-revenue activities that contribute to your practice's success

Savvy practitioners know that success requires more than a certain number of patients and a certain amount of generated income—it also requires goodwill within your community. If your associates speak to kennel clubs and school groups, for example, they help generate long-term goodwill for the practice while lowering your long-term marketing costs.

I've seen some veterinarians in group practices, however, who generate high personal gross income from an overflow of clients cultivated by their associates, who spend exhaustive hours in the exam room and out in the community building such goodwill.

Therefore, associates who participate in goodwill-building activities deserve a higher percentage of their personal production. In general, this factor will raise or lower compensation no more than one to two percent; but combined with other factors, the increase could make a considerable difference both in salary and job satisfaction.

Complex ... but worth it

Some practice owners are concerned that compensation based on production will lead associates to perform unnecessary procedures to pad the bill. My response: No! Associates face no greater inclination to pad the bill than practice owners. Remember, owner veterinarians always work for compensation based on   production ... it's called net income! Associate compensation is a complex issue; but before you throw up your hands and say, "Why bother?" consider this: When compensation is based on productivity, individual production and personal satisfaction almost always increase. Most important, associate veterinarians begin to behave like practice owners, which results in improved client satisfaction.

Blended compensation

By Ross Clark, DVM

Experienced practice owners of the '70s and '80s, along with practice management consultants, had all pretty much accepted as a general rule that associates with five or more years of experience receive up to two times the salaries paid new graduates. But my experience, confirmed by *Veterinary Economics* surveys, indicates that in the mid '90s, senior veterinarian salaries are currently only 1.55 times those of new graduates.

Why the lower number? I'm confident that it's because computers have enabled practice managers to measure individual productivity more accurately. In addition, computers have enhanced the productivity of new graduates by eliminating the majority of fee-reduction opportunities. By leveling the productivity playing field, experience may no longer ensure senior veterinarians' double production levels—or double salaries. Practice owners, however, may continue to award higher salaries to experienced doctors for the non-monetary contributions they make to the practice.

The table shown here provides guidelines for a guaranteed base salary plus compensation based on individual production. The figures refer to 1992 data and are based on the following assumptions: A veterinarian working 45 hours a week works 195 hours a month and 2,340 hours per year. Subtracting 150 hours for vacation, sick leave and holidays leaves the doctor working 2,190 hours a year (182.5 a month) to generate the necessary income to cover his or her expected salary. I recommend an additional eight to 10 percent of personal production in excess of expected production.

A new graduate expecting $30,000 at 20 percent of gross must then generate $150,000 individual gross income annually, which is $12,500 per month, or $68.49 per hour. The experienced veterinarian expecting a $46,500 annual salary at 20 percent of gross must generate $19,375 individual gross income per month—or $106.16 per hour.

The table assumes an average of two and a half full-time equivalent support staff per veterinarian. Keep in mind that salaries must be adjusted to consider local supply and demand for veterinarians, the local cost of living index, volume of clients, variance

Years of experience	Annual salary	Monthly salary	Expected monthly production	Expected annual production
0-1	$30,000	$2,500	$12,500	$150,000
1-2	33,300	2,775	13,875	166,500
2-3	36,300	3,025	15,125	181,500
3-4	39,900	3.325	16,625	199,500
4-5	43,200	3,600	18,000	216,000
5 or more	46,500	3,875	19,375	232,500

in hours worked and total number of support staff per veterinarian, regardless of the method of compensation used.

Blended form of compensation

Using the chart above you may want to award to associate veterinarians a bonus of eight to 10 percent of their individual production above their expected monthly production. Example: A new graduate in the Midwest is paid an annual salary of $30,000 and has an expected monthly production of $12,500. If this veterinarian should have a month of only $11,000 production, there is no penalty and the veterinarian receives a full salary. If the veterinarian has a production of $14,000, then he or she would be due a bonus of $150 ($1,500 x 10 percent).

Partnership agreements

by Ross D. Clark, DVM, and David Madden, JD, attorney in Overland Park, Kan.

A partnership agreement is one of the most important contracts you will use in your practice. In my practice, the partnership agreement keeps each partner current as to his or her financial returns and hospital work responsibilities, both clinical and managerial. It leaves little, if anything, to doubt. It also prevents the development of bitter feelings that might result from misunderstood expectations.

I have provided a model partnership agreement in the accompanying *Practice Workbook,* Section 3: Contracts, that will assist you in shaping your own contract. That sample agreement contains numerous items you should consider including in your own contract. But first, here are some helpful comments:

Before selecting the appropriate business structure—partnership or corporation—the veterinarian should consider the legal and financial consequences of each form of practice. The veterinarian should know what personal liability will result from the business structure he or she selects for his or her practice. If the veterinarian engages in a partnership, is his or her liability individual or joint? It is often said that a businessman can escape personal liability by incorporation. But in those states that permit professional corporations, the professional is not allowed to escape individual liability for his or her negligence; and, for the most part, his or her creditors will require both corporate and individual liability.

Finally, anyone selecting a business structure should carefully weigh the tax aspects of this business. Anyone entering into a partnership should realize that it is a legal relationship and a personal relationship. It is much like a marriage. Its termination can be as disastrous financially and emotionally as a divorce.

We recommend that written agreements be made prior to setting up a business relationship. A partnership is a contract; the parties forming one must be capable of entering into contractual relations. As with any business, a partnership will have a name, accumulate property and have profits and losses. The written partnership agreement must address these issues.

Many states have passed the Uniform Partnership Act and Limited Liability Partnership Act. These Acts define the partnership relationship and set out a statutory scheme for answering questions that arise in the course of the partnership. The Limited Liability Partnership Act can "limit" the exposure of partners in certain situations. You should consult legal counsel to ensure that any written partnership agreement into which you enter complies with the law of the state in which you practice.

If a veterinarian enters into a general partnership, that partnership should have a written agreement that at a minimum:

- Sets out a plan for determining the ownership of property brought into the partnership, property purchased after the formation of the partnership and the distribution of property in the event of a dissolution of the partnership;

- Describes a means for the division of profits and losses;

- Defines the liabilities of the parties as to one another;

- Defines the rights and duties of the parties; and

- Provides for an orderly dissolution of the partnership in the event of the admission of a new partner, withdrawal or retirement of a partner and the death or disability of a partner.

How many times have you heard a partnership compared to a marriage, with divorce possibly down the road? Probably too often. That metaphor is so common now that it really fails to carry its true impact. However, partnerships *can* involve marriages. Recently, I consulted at two practices where the partners were husband and wife veterinarians. Unfortunately, they had not drawn up partnership agreements. Then divorce struck, and the couples were fighting in court over what to do with their practice. In one case, both the husband and wife wanted the practice. In the other instance, neither one wanted the practice or its staggering liabilities.

In some ways many practices involve marriages, but usually the spouse of the practitioner is not a veterinarian. That spouse, however, in the event of divorce can force the practice into difficult circumstances, such as sale.

How do you guard against the unforeseen, the unlikely? It's not easy. Whether or not your practice involves just you and your spouse or other practitioners, you need some sort of insurance to keep your interests safe and everyone from gunning each other down.

Your partnership agreement can be your insurance policy against disaster. One of the most important parts of this agreement provides for the distribution of the practice assets in case one of the dreadful four Ds occurs: disagreement, disability, death or divorce. What would you do if your partner walked in one day and said he had to sell his half of the practice to pay off a divorce settlement? Without a clear agreement, you have no way to protect your interest in the practice.

*Author's note: A Limited Liability Partnership contract should also be considered.

Chapter 8:
Leasing, Buying and Selling Practices

Negotiating leases

by Ross D. Clark, DVM

As a practice management consultant, I have always been surprised by the number of veterinarians who enter lease agreements between senior and junior partners without proper legal documentation. A lease is one of the most common legal agreements you'll encounter in your career. You may begin as a lessee, either as part of a practice corporation leasing from the senior partner or as a practice owner leasing space in a shopping center. Later in your career, you may own a freestanding facility, leasing to yourself and others in a veterinary practice partnership.

A lease is a conveyance of an interest in real property. Historically, it has been referred to as a limited estate. In real property law, there are basically two kinds of interest grants in real estate: fee simple and fee determinable, or limited. When you receive a fee simple grant, as when you purchase a home, you receive all rights to the property. A lease is a limited grant of the use of real property. Essentially, a lease is a contract to use specific real property for a specific purpose. Concepts of real property law and contract law are applied to the drafting, enforcement and interpretation of a lease. There are two kinds of leases: commercial and residential.

Whether you're the lessee or the lessor, you should be sure that your lease agreement spells out all the pertinent details. Here are the major points to consider when negotiating a lease.

Length of the lease

How long should a lease be in effect? To determine the answer for your situation, ask yourself this question: Is the leased space going to be your permanent location or do you plan to move or build somewhere else? Your decision may be swayed by the rental rate. If the rent is reasonable, you may want to secure that low rate for future years.

When you've determined how long the lease will run, establish when it begins. Unless the space is vacant and already remodeled to fit your needs, you can run into all sorts of problems. Sometimes an old tenant will refuse to move out; construction may not be finished on time; disagreements may arise about whether you can gain early access to install fixtures or make your own improvements.

To avoid such problems, make sure your lease agreement clearly details what happens if the space isn't ready and what adjustments will be made to compensate. Be wary of a clause stipulating that the landlord will provide an alternate space if yours isn't ready; such a clause makes that possibility more likely. And, as you know, it's not feasible for a veterinary hospital to move in and set up shop somewhere else for just a few months.

When a lease expires, the landlord has no obligation to renew it—unless you've agreed on a renewal formula and have a written clause that gives you first rights to the space when your lease runs out. Without these stipulations, you may end up paying the market rate to stay on, or you may be forced to leave. If you plan to make your leased space a permanent site for your practice, get a renewal agreement to ensure security and to help plan for future rental costs. A fair way to adjust renewal rental rates is to tie them to the local consumer price index.

I know of one veterinarian that negotiated for six months at "no rent" for signing a five-year lease with a renewal option (tied to inflation) every five years for the next 25 years.

Cost of rent

Landlords base the rent they charge on one of several types of leases. The leases you might encounter include:

- *Gross lease:* The tenant is required to pay a flat monthly rate, and the landlord is responsible for paying all of the operating expenses. In the past, these expenses have included utilities; but because of rising energy costs, those likely will no longer be included.

- *Net lease:* In addition to the base rent, the tenant is responsible for providing payment for some or all of the real estate taxes owed on the building.

- *Double-net lease:* In addition to rent and taxes, the tenant pays for insurance on the space that he rents.

- *Triple-net lease:* The tenant is responsible for paying all of the operating expenses of the space he or she rents, including the taxes, insurance and utilities.

- *Percentage lease:* This is a special type of lease designed for retailers in shopping malls. It requires that the tenant pay a percentage of gross income in addition to a base rent.

Most lessors provide repair service to the building for such things as air conditioning, heating, electricity, plumbing and water heaters. Care of the parking lot and grounds around the building usually are the responsibility of the building owner. Most shopping malls and strip centers, however, charge a monthly maintenance fee.

Most landlords carry insurance on the building, but they have the right to insist that their tenants carry their own insurance to protect them from civil claims that might arise. It's also a good idea to check your policy and your landlord's policy to make sure you are covered in case of theft or fire.

Location, size

The right location is vital to the success of your clinic. When selecting a lease site, you'll want to know such things as the population and household income of the surrounding neighborhoods. A demographic study can help you compile and analyze these statistics.

> *The right location is vital to the success of your clinic. When selecting a lease site, you'll want to know such things as the population and household income of the surrounding neighborhoods.*

When checking over a lease, be sure it allows you to put up your "shingle" and, if you're in a strip mall, that your business will appear on the mall's marquee. Also check to be sure that the number of parking spaces available for your exclusive use will be sufficient.

One of the most common complaints I encounter is that leasing offers very limited opportunities for veterinarians to expand. But that doesn't have to be the case. Opportunity for growth is an essential factor to consider before you lease, particularly if you plan to lease a space for a great length of time. Be sure your lease allows such growth. In the event that empty space becomes available, you should have first right of refusal. If you plan to do some remodeling, do some rough drawings to make sure there is enough space for everything you want to include.

Improvements

One topic often overlooked when negotiating a lease is improvements. The questions you need to ask are: Who pays for the improvements? Can you take them with you when you move? Are there any guidelines that need to be followed when making improvements, such as the type of wall coverings and floor coverings allowed?

I know veterinarians who have designed and built their cabinets, reception counters and exam tables so that they could take them along when they moved to a freestanding hospital.

You also should pay close attention to the overall quality of the building. How soundproof are the walls? What type of lighting is available, and how much? Provided your lease allows, you can improve existing conditions. Remember, though, that it's probably less expensive and less time-consuming to choose a rental space that closely fits your needs and requires only minor changes to finish the job. One key is to pick a space at the end of a strip shopping center; then put your kennel room next to the outside wall. This reduces the chance of noise complaints by at least 75 percent.

Security

Besides your expensive equipment and drug inventory, you're in charge of pets whose owners place their trust in you and in the safety of your building. Be sure that some sort of security is ensured by your lease. Take into consideration parking lot lighting and neighborhood business activity late at night.

Although security for the building is usually the responsibility of the owner, you *can* take added measures. You might, for example, consider investing in a security patrol, alarm system or a guard dog. Make sure the lease allows you to provide additional security and that whatever you use can be taken with you when you decide to leave.

Neighbors, competition

Because of the unique nature of veterinary medicine, some business owners might take exception to having you as a neighbor. Make sure you are protected from requests by your neighbors that you move out because you're disrupting their business. One veterinarian I know has a lease that states that if someone moves in next to him and then complains about the noise or the smell of the clinic, then that person, not the veterinarian, has to leave. And don't forget competition from another veterinary hospital or a pet store that might move into the shopping mall. Make an exclusivity agreement with your landlord before this problem arises.

Lawyers

Finally, it's a good idea to ask a lawyer to draw up the lease to make sure it is a legal and enforceable document in your state. If you choose to draw up your own lease or accept the landlord's lease, at least take it to a lawyer and let him or her check it over for mistakes or oversights.

People generally do not read lease agreements; and if they do read them, they do not always understand them. A lease is a contract that defines the rights and duties of the lessor and lessee. Any prospective landlord or renter should be sure to include all the terms for which they have bargained in their lease. Lawyers commonly see the problems of interpretation with leases. Remember, the basic rule of law is that the lease is most strongly interpreted in favor of the non-drafting party in the event of an honest question of interpretation.

Other factors

Another item to be considered in leases is the use of escalation clauses to protect the lessor from the vagaries of inflation.

In addition, the lease should provide for a landlord's lien upon the lessee's property contained in the leased premises in the event the lessee defaults in payment of the rent.

Other clauses to consider include those concerning the right to exhibit the premises, subrogation, security deposit and subordination to mortgage. There is no single form that will precisely fit each situation; however, the example shown in the accompanying *Pracice Workbook,* Section 3: Contracts, reflects the minimal considerations necessary in drawing a lease between a prospective tenant and a landlord.

Buying and selling practices

by Ross D. Clark, DVM, and Ron Patrick, CPA

Whether buyers or sellers, the people involved in a practice sale want to achieve certain goals in the transaction. A buyer wants to finance the price, but a seller may prefer all cash. A buyer wants to be sure the net receipts will cover all bills and allow a comfortable income, but a seller may want to be sure there is ample security to replace the cash flow. Each party wants something a little different. That is why it is important for both parties to be as knowledgeable as possible before entering into any buy-sell arrangement.

Buyers must understand that several different factors are involved in buying a practice. They must select the right practice–paying particular attention to location. They must also know what combination of assets they are purchasing: inventory, equipment, real estate, improvements, goodwill and client records.

Both parties, especially the seller, need to examine the liabilities and tax considerations. Restrictive practice covenants must be negotiated. All of these factors must be reviewed before any kind of buying decision is made.

Buying a practice

Selecting the right practice: Anyone in real estate will confirm that the first three principles of the trade are *location, location and location*. These three principles must be used when selecting the right practice.

An existing practice is committed to its location, which can make it a little vulnerable. As a buyer, one needs to know what factors affect the right location.

Residential areas: Choose a practice in a city, or part of a city, that seems to be experiencing population growth. Better yet, search for a practice that is located on a road servicing a popular residential area. Convenience is very important. Most clients do not like taking their pets long distances in a car.

Exposure and accessibility: In most cases, a freestanding clinic has better exposure than a shopping center clinic. Parking is often better, and location is nearer the street. Shopping center clinics, however, often attract clients who are visiting other shops in the center. A good compromise is a location in a neighborhood convenience center. Consider, by way of example, a practice in Tulsa that had been practicing in the Briarglen Village shopping center for eight or nine years. In September of 1994, Dr. Jeff Schoenhals moved the practice to a street-frontage property 300 feet away and around the corner from the center, and the number of new clients doubled from 30 per month to 60 per month–a sizable increase for a solo practice. Assuming these 30 new clients averaged 1.6 pets and 2.5 visits per year at $50 per visit, the potential increased gross for this practice increased by $72,000 per year (1.6 x 2.5 x $50 x 30 = $6,000/month x 12 = $72,000/year) due to that 300-foot move.

Household count

Survey the neighborhoods surrounding the practice and try to estimate whether there are more single-family or multiple-family (apartments and condominiums) dwellings. Pet restrictions often apply to multiple-family dwellings and that would limit the client base. Choose a location near mostly single-family homes. Across America, about 52 percent of households have either a dog or cat. When all pets are considered, 61 percent of households have dogs, cats, birds, hamsters or horses.

Draw three-, five- and 10-mile circles around the proposed practice site, and count the veterinarians within each circle. Divide the total number of veterinarians into the number of households within the circle. Studies indicate that a practice needs a potential client base of at least 1,500 pets. Therefore, each veterinarian would need a minimum of 2,000 households (a population of approximately 5,000) that use veterinary medical services.

Those households having pets will each have an average of 1.6 pets. In more affluent neighborhoods, as many as 85 percent of all households will seek veterinary medical services. In less affluent neighborhoods, less than 50 percent may seek veterinary services.

Assuming 50 percent of households have 1.5 pets and 66 percent will seek veterinary medical services, we would like to see 3,000 households per veterinarian in the three areas chosen. Of that 3,000, probably 1,500 households will have pets. Two-thirds (1,000) of those households will seek veterinary services.

In 1,000 households, there will be about 1,500 pets. Assuming a comprehensive practice can gross $140 per pet per year (the national average is $80 per year), then this practice location would have a potential gross of $210,000 per year.

Of course, some practices succeed with demographics that are not as favorable as those suggested here; and others fail with demographics better than these. Just be aware that increased competition may soon change the demographic ground rules. National corporate-financed practices are having an impact on practice growth. (See Chapter 4: Marketing, advertising and public relations for additional information on marketing.)

Household income

The mean income of an area is another indicator of potential revenue for a practice. Search for a middle-income neighborhood, or higher, with a large number of school-aged children. Enrollment records from community schools can provide this information unless private schools or busing are factors. Look for the community's personal income to total at least $95 million per veterinarian.

Traffic count

Clients need easy access to a practice. A practice located on a major six-lane highway with a center median and no access may attract less business than a practice on a two-lane road with easy access. And remember those intersections: When traffic slows down, drivers notice the practice more easily.

Setting the right price

Once the practice and its location have been evaluated, the next step is to establish a price. Both buyer and seller need to value the tangible and intangible assets of the practice. Tangibles include inventory, equipment, real estate and improvements. Intangibles include goodwill and client records.

Inventory: Included in the inventory are items held for resale (e.g., prescription diets, vitamins, flea sprays, topicals) and single items held for hospital use (e.g., injectables). These items are usually priced at replacement cost.

Price adjustments should be made for partially used or damaged items. The buyer should review the items to see whether anything is incompatible with the new practice. For example, if the seller stocks drugs used for large animals but the buyer intends to practice only on small animals, he or she may not want to purchase the large-animal items.

The actual inventory varies daily, so the inventory list should be prepared on the closing date of the sale. During negotiations, estimates are used. On the final inventory, the buyer should perform or at least observe inventory audit.

When taking the inventory, be systematic to avoid deletions or duplications. Start at one end of the clinic and count all items in a room. If a particular item is in more than one room, list all the items found in that room and then add in similar items from other rooms. During the physical count, one person should list the items and another should count the items. The inventory team can self-check its counts and can also note the condition of items.

Equipment: The practice's equipment should be listed just like inventory. This category includes large and small medical equipment (e.g., instruments, office furniture, fixtures, vehicles, cages, computers and anything else that is not permanently affixed to the building or land.)

Equipment is valued differently than inventory. Inventory is normally sold or used within a short period after purchase, but equipment may last for years. One method for valuing equipment is "discounted replacement cost." This method values an item at what it would cost to replace it, less any loss in value as its useful life decreases.

In other words, it assumes all equipment will be used only a certain number of years. As time passes, the remaining useful life becomes shorter, so the method reduces the replacement cost of the equipment proportional to its remaining useful life.

This method is especially useful for medical equipment and other items of limited marketability. Office equipment can be valued by using the cost of comparable used equipment. As with inventory, review the equipment list for obsolete items or items that are not needed. Our company, Veterinary Management Concepts (Appraisal Division), usually uses 75 percent of current replacement cost.

Real estate and improvements: If real estate is included in a sale, it should be valued by an independent real estate appraiser. Be sure to select someone who is familiar with the practice's location and the local economy. Appraisers often value property differently, so a second or third opinion is a good idea. Ask for an abbreviated (drive-by) appraisal for negotiation purposes.

If the practice is located on leased property, the seller must place a value on the lease and improvements. If the rent is below the rental value of the property, the lease has value to the buyer. But if the rent is above the rental value, the lease is actually a liability and the purchase price should be reduced accordingly. One way to adjust a lease is to multiply the difference between actual rent payments and fair rental value by the number of months remaining in the lease. The result is the adjustment (up or down) in the selling price.

Goodwill: The goodwill of a practice is the value of its past business and its accumulation of clients, hired employees and start-up activities necessary for any new business. It can be valued simply or derived from complicated formulas. Whatever the method, when placing value on goodwill, one should consider the current condition of the practice. Potential improvements are left to the buyer and cannot add any value for the seller.

One simple method of valuing goodwill is as a percentage of one year's gross income. The percentage could vary from 50 to 125 percent of one year's gross income, depending on practice age, condition and demographic trends. Gross income would be the weighted average of the last three years' cash receipts from services and product sales, with most emphasis on the last year if the practice is growing.

Under this method, goodwill would be the amount left over after subtracting the value of inventory, equipment and other assets (excluding real estate). Rule-of-thumb methods can be very easy—and very wrong!

Another simple method is to negotiate a value for each patient record and then buy the records at their negotiated value. This is an especially good method if the practice will be relocated or merged into an existing practice, because the newly purchased practice will lose its identity and its only intangible value will be its client base.

An example of the formula method is the Owen E. McCafferty/ *Veterinary Economics* formula for evaluation of a practice. This method adjusts the net income of the practice by adding back unusual or personal expenses and subtracting normal expenses that a new owner would expect to incur. From this adjusted net income, fair salary for veterinarians is subtracted as a fair amount for the cost to the buyer. Any amount left over is capitalized over a three- to six-year period. The underlying assumption in this method is that goodwill is only present if the net income exceeds certain normal expectations, including fair salary and fair rent to the owner veterinarian(s). It is difficult to apply this method to new practices because of the lack of historical data.

As was mentioned earlier, employees are also part of a practice's "goodwill" value. The buyer "purchases" these individuals' talents and expertise. Existing employees can have intrinsic value because they are acquainted with the clients and they are trained, which frees the buyer's time for other business activities. Existing employees also work together as a team, which can help smooth rough transitional time. In some cases, however, the buyer may decide that the existing staff is a liability; in which case, the goodwill figure should be adjusted accordingly.

Client or patient records: A quick method of calculating patient records is to count all the patient records whose owners' names begin with "S." Multiply this total by 10 to arrive at the estimated total number of patients. (Note: If the hospital in question keeps more than one patient on each client's card, it is important to multiply the number of client cards by 1.6 to get the total number of patients.)

A court case in California in 1977 determined that veterinary medical records do have value. At that time, the U.S. Internal Revenue Service accepted $7.50 per record as a proper value. In 1995, $25 to $30 was a fair value, depending, of course, on the annual gross per patient.

The gross per patient can be calculated by dividing the total current records (all clients who have been in at least one time in the last 36 months) into the annual gross. Our studies indicate $85 per pet per year is average. A gross of $200 per pet per year would justify a higher value per record. Client records can be depreciated over a seven-year period.

Liability: Normally, the buyer does not assume any old liabilities; the seller pays them. The buyer might, however, inadvertently become liable when purchasing shares of stock in an existing corporation. The corporation is usually liable for all debts, regardless of change in ownership.

Another potential problem is that one might buy assets without knowing there are liens that exist against those assets. Ask the seller about debts owed and to whom they are owed. Then call the creditor to be sure the liens are released.

The buyer may also specify that a portion of the purchase price be held in escrow (with interest accruing to the seller) for a certain period of time to handle any liabilities or claims that may be asserted against the practice. Whatever the plan of action, the buyer must be sure to clear any unnecessary debt.

Tax considerations: Many details of the sale can result in conflict between the tax situations of the buyer and the seller.

Example 1:

If a buyer pays a seller $100,000 for an existing veterinary practice to be allocated as follows:

Inventory	$10,000
Equipment	$60,000
Goodwill	$30,000
Total	$100,000

Then the $30,000 goodwill could result in favorable capital gains tax treatment to the seller.

Example 2:

If, however, the $100,000 were justifiably allocated as follows:

Inventory	$10,000
Equipment	$90,000
Goodwill	$ 0
Total	$100,000

Then the buyer would be able to depreciate the higher equipment value and receive a tax deduction more quickly. The seller might have to recapture a greater portion of depreciation as ordinary income.

Remember: Medical records are now subject to a 15-year amortization period.

Another tax consideration is how the purchase price of the practice will be paid. If it is paid all in the same year, the seller may be forced into a higher tax bracket. By spreading payments over two or more years, this might be avoided or at least mitigated.

The transfer of titles to assets may be structured to obtain maximum tax benefit without affecting the negotiations process. If the buyer plans to operate the practice as a corporation, more might be saved by holding some assets personally and transferring others to the corporation. The personal assets could be leased to the corporation. The corporation would receive deductions for rent payments, and the new owner could report the rent as income. The new owner would then receive depreciation deductions on the assets to partially or wholly offset the rent income. The net result is that the corporation receives a tax deduction and the new owner can take money out of the corporation without being subjected to income or payroll taxes.

A non-tax-related reason for not transferring all assets to the new practice is that the buyer thus retains control of those assets. As new veterinarians are allowed to buy into the practice in the future, either as partners or as shareholders, the personally held assets are unaffected. This results in a lower purchase price for the new veterinarians and lets the senior partner maintain control of some of the assets.

Tax planning should be an integral part of the negotiation process. Seek competent tax advice before finalizing any sale because tax laws are complex and change continually.

Restrictive practice covenants

Any buyer is rightfully nervous about the seller's plans once the agreement is consummated. What prevents the seller from moving a couple of blocks down the street, hanging out his or her shingle and "stealing" all those dearly purchased clients the buyer has just acquired as part of the practice's goodwill? The restrictive practice covenant helps solve this problem.

A restrictive practice covenant helps the buyer become established in the marketplace without competition from the seller. The covenant, written into the final agreement, places limitations on the seller. The buyer would want to limit the location where the seller may practice in the future or set a particular number of years before the seller can practice again in the area. A typical urban practice could justify 10 miles for five years.

The only problem with restrictive covenants is their enforcement. Even though agreements in all 50 states may include such clauses, some lawyers argue that restrictive covenants are illegal because a person's right to make a living cannot be limited in certain extenuating circumstances.

Still, be sure to include the clause for as much protection as possible. When money is paid for goodwill, it has been this author's observations that covenants not to compete are almost always enforceable.

Selling a practice

The value of a practice is the amount somebody is willing to sell it for and someone else is willing to pay for it. Many veterinarians, however, sell their practices too cheaply. If you find yourself in the seller's seat, try following these guidelines well in advance to come out ahead.

Time: The seller should plan ahead to allow plenty of time to prepare for the sale. Some business brokers recommend up to five years of planning. Why so long? Long-range planning provides the seller a chance to build the practice into a salable item as well as time to prepare for a career change, retirement or transfer.

Annual appraisals: Have the practice evaluated yearly, especially when you have a partnership or corporation with multiple veterinarians. This will help you accurately chart your progress. Being able to show the internal or external buyer what has been done to increase the worth of the business over the past five to seven years will aid in negotiations. If you can demonstrate that the practice is growing, you can negotiate a higher price. Most appraisal firms will have a somewhat reduced rate for these annual appraisals.

Growth curves: The seller should monitor increases in growth as well as in value. Demonstrate with a graph how the patient load has increased. Note the peak and slump times of the year. Show the impact of fee increases on receipts. Illustrate the impact of adding a new partner or technician.

Improvements: Building improvements should also be documented. For the most part, stick to paint and other surface changes. Big changes may not be appreciated by the buyer, and the increased rent or price may make the practice too expensive to the buyer. Decide what kinds of improvements would increase the value of the business without overpricing it. These improvements can be taken as depreciation benefits while increasing the value of the property for the upcoming sale.

Cash flow: Finally, go all out to strengthen the practice's cash flow. Each dollar brought to the bottom line is multiplied by an average capitalization rate of five. Be sure the financial statement is as sound as possible. The seller's banker, the buyer and the buyer's banker will be impressed; and the seller will be able to walk away from the sale with more money in his or her pocket.

Establish a price: Review the guidelines outlined above on price setting. Complete the inventory and establish the value of the equipment. Know the worth of the real estate and improvements. Determine a price for goodwill and client records. When the seller has accounted every item of value and has given it a fair yet marketable value, he or she is then ready to look for a buyer.

Look within

When selling, look within the practice first. If the seller knows the buyer and they have worked together for a few years, the buyer can feel more confident that the practice will run smoothly after the seller is gone and the seller is more assured of receiving any rental payments or note payments that are due.

This is where planning comes in. When sellers know they want to retire or move within five years, they should offer the practice to a current associate who is interested in buying a practice down the road—or *hire* such an associate. Then, the seller and the potential buyer know each other and will have a chance to change plans in case the relationship does not work out. Potential buyers benefit because the clientele gets to know them, which helps to ensure a smoother transition when the seller leaves the practice.

Gradual buy/sell method

The gradual buy/sell method lets the eventual seller (the senior veterinarian/owner) benefit from the buyer's (junior veterinarian's) additional income by increasing the senior's income. Junior associates benefit by deducting a portion of client records and equipment from their income tax. For example: A young veterinarian has an opportunity to buy into a growing practice and will be paying little or nothing down. Both parties can benefit in this type of arrangement. The new partnership pays the junior partner, who has acquired one percent to 50 percent of the practice, a fair wage based on experience (see Chapter 7: Partnership and associate agreements, "Associate compensation" and "Blended compensation") plus a percentage of profits after all expenses have been paid (including a fair wage to all veterinarians and fair building rent). As an example, the junior partner makes $100 more and the senior partner, therefore, takes home $100 less. That saves the senior partner $38 in taxes based on a 38-percent tax rate. The junior partner pays taxes on his additional $100 at his 15-percent tax bracket. Then he pays the $100 back to the senior partner in the form of a note. The senior partner pays capital gains taxes on the $100 because he has sold part of an asset.

Put another way, the senior partner gives the junior partner $100 additional income and receives the money back in the form of capital gain when the junior associate makes his note payment. Income tax advantages for both parties help make the transaction even more worthwhile. Another advantage for the junior associate is that he or she can deduct a portion of client records and equipment from income taxes. The junior partner can depreciate client records and equipment over seven years. So for that $25,000 in assets purchased, he or she can depreciate roughly $3,500 in each of the seven years.

Negotiable items

Naturally, the buyer and seller have different goals in the purchase, but there is room for negotiation. Purchase price is only one area.

The purchase price depends on other factors, such as the down payment, the interest rate and the term, which is in turn affected by the age of the seller. If the buyer must finance the purchase price, that price goes up because the seller is now losing money that could be earning income or interest elsewhere. Both parties have to be willing to give and take so they can arrive at a compromise.

Another area for negotiation is old inventory. The practice may have inventory that will probably sell, but the items may not sell for a year or more. These could be special-order items that were returned or never picked up or items that just do not move quickly. The seller can offer that merchandise at a price lower than its replacement cost to compensate for the long holding period.

Buy-out agreements

Buy-out agreements have the following objectives:

- To restrict transferability of ownership interest to unknown parties;
- To give either the entity or the other owners an option or duty to purchase the business interest upon the occurrence of certain specified events (e.g., retirement, permanent disability, death);
- To provide a covenant not to compete;
- To provide estate liquidity;
- To provide financial support for the spouse of a deceased owner veterinarian;
- To avoid having executors or conservators become owners of business interest;
- To fix the value of business interest for federal estate tax purpose.

Methods of funding the buy-out include:

- Life Insurance;
- Disability Insurance.

Closing the deal

When the buyer and seller have settled on a price, negotiated the terms and agreed to follow through with the transaction, it is time to close the deal. Be sure to draw up the appropriate documents from those listed here:

- Partnership agreement, if applicable (see Chapter 7: Partnership and associate agreements, "Partnership agreements").

- A promissory note from the purchasing partner and his executors, administrators and heirs. The debtor assigns and guarantees payment to the seller, his administrators and his heirs (if applicable).

- A purchase agreement.

- Collateral pledge, if applicable.

- Equipment lease agreement for tax purposes, if applicable. (The buying partner might buy, under a separate agreement, a percentage of the oldest equipment. This could be in addition to the portion of the practice purchase. The buying partner can then "re-depreciate" this equipment. Each partner in turn leases his or her equipment to the partnership/seller, could "gift" all or part of existing equipment to his children, and the new partnership could lease equipment from children. Again, check current tax legislation to learn whether this is beneficial.)

- Real estate lease agreement, if applicable.

There are four major areas where both parties can seek professional guidance:

- Finding a buyer or seller,
- Setting the purchase price,
- Tax planning and
- Obtaining legal services

Finding a buyer or seller

Often the buyer and seller find each other without too much searching. The seller may be a retiring partner who is selling his share, and the buyer may be an employee being offered a partnership interest. Many times, though, the buyer and seller may need a third party to get them together. They can turn to a practice broker for help.

Practice brokers are much like real estate brokers in that they contact sellers and buyers and charge a fee for this service–usually a percentage of the sales price.

The broker can help the seller determine a reasonable asking price for the practice and can offer suggestions that may make the practice more attractive to a prospective buyer. The broker will also actively promote the seller's practice and search for buyers.

Remember that a broker represents the seller's interests. A prospective buyer should listen to a broker's sales pitch with caution.

Setting the purchase price

There are two primary considerations to setting a purchase price. One is an objective appraisal of the practice's assets, liabilities and goodwill; the other is the negotiations.

The appraisal: This is usually performed by someone hired by either the buyer, the seller or both. The independent appraiser values the business using objective sources such as tax returns or audited financial statements, physical counts and inventories and industry information. The appraiser should not be biased toward either the buyer or the seller.

If you are the seller and you use an accountant, be sure to use a firm with experience in veterinary practice sales. I believe that accounting firms with experience only in the human and dental fields tend to undervalue veterinary practices by 25 to 40 percent. When a veterinarian dies or retires, the practice location and value tend to transfer very well. When a physician or dentist dies, the practice tends to die with them; the one exception being group practice.

The appraisal firms that I know as the largest and most experienced in America are:

O.E.M. Associates
Cleveland, OH

Simmons and Associates, Inc.
1610-A Frederica Rd.
St. Simons Island, GA 31522-2509

Stuart J. Yasgoor, PC
Suite 310
500 Sepulveda Blvd.
Los Angeles, CA 90049

And our firm ...
Appraisal Division
Veterinary Management Concepts, Inc.
Suite A
4720 East 51st Street
Tulsa, OK 74135

The negotiations: Another aspect of setting a purchase price is the negotiator. Someone needs to get the best price, terms and conditions for whomever they represent. An attorney could rep-

negotiator for the seller.

Both of these phases are critical to ensure that a practice is sold as quickly as possible and that each party receives fair treatment. Professional fees are minimal compared with the cost of a mistake.

Tax planning

Normally the results of tax planning will not change the basic sales agreement. What it may change are the structure, timing and method of the sale. Buyers and sellers can have conflicting desires when it comes to tax planning. Therefore, both parties must know all the consequences of the sale. Both the buyer and the seller should hire their own tax advisor and consult him or her before finalizing the agreement.

Legal services

This is yet another area where each party should have its own counsel. An attorney advocates his or her client and should not be expected to do anything but maximize that client's position.

The attorney draws up the proper documents and provides advice on how to structure the sale to avoid costly legal problems in the future; so always obtain legal assistance before finalizing any terms or conditions. Remember: In community property states, don't overlook spousal interest in the practice.

In the event of dissolution of an owner's marriage, the agreement should require the active spouse to obtain full control of the business interest; and, if this is not done, the other owners should have an enforceable option to purchase the nonactive spouse's interest. In the event of death of the active spouse, the community property interest of the nonactive spouse should specifically be included in the buy-out rights.

Summary

Both buyer and seller should educate themselves before entering into any kind of agreement.

The buyer should research the practice and try to evaluate its value, learn whether there are outstanding liabilities and examine the tax considerations.

Sellers should plan well in advance of the venture, establish an equitable price and try to sell to someone they know.

As the deal is closed, negotiate items to arrive at a compromise; be sure to include all the necessary documentation.

All parties should seek professional help.

If buyers and sellers follow these guidelines, the sale or purchase of a practice will be smoother and less troublesome.

Sources:

Clark, R., and R. K. Patrick. "How to buy or sell a practice." *Veterinary Practice Management.* D.M. McCurnin, editor. Philadelphia: Lippincott Medical Publishing, 1988: 138-158.

Judy, J. Michigan State University. Personal Communication.

McCafferty, O. E. "How to price your practice (Parts I, II, III)." *Veterinary Economics.* July 1983: 38-51; August 1983: 56-64; September 1983: 68-70.

Yasgoor, S. J. "Buying an equity interest in an existing veterinary practice." Western Veterinary Conference. February 20, 1991.

Eight creative strategies for financing a practice

By Ross Clark, DVM

Far too many veterinary practice sales fall through because the buyer and seller can't agree on financing. Here's a typical scenario: You're ready to buy a practice, but you can't swing the hefty closing costs the seller requires. You can re-negotiate, but that's likely to leave you with too little cash and too large a debt—and leave the seller with a reduced selling price. Of course, another option is to forget about the deal altogether. But either way, you both lose.

But financing problems don't have to destroy the sale of a veterinary practice. Don't give up on a deal until you've considered all of your financing options. With a little creativity, you can save the sale with a deal that pleases both the buyer and the seller. The key is for both parties to define their objectives openly; then develop a plan to meet those objectives. With an open mind, financing opportunities are virtually unlimited. Here are eight creative strategies to smooth the sale of a veterinary practice.

1. Sell excess assets.

If you are the buyer, you should review the practice's asset lists to determine if there are items you won't need. Say the hospital has a retiring partner who has practiced only a minimal amount of time in the past two years. The practice may have maintained extra equipment that will be unnecessary with a smaller staff. You may be able to sell the extra equipment and use the cash proceeds toward the down payment.

2. Ask the seller to keep some assets.

You can ask the seller if he or she will keep accounts receivable, thereby reducing the purchase price and the required down payment. If the seller refuses, try to sell the accounts receivable or borrow against them at a discount. This discount may prove expensive; but in an emergency, you'll have a ready source of cash.

You also can ask the seller to reduce the inventory level specified in the price, then apply the difference to the down payment.

3. Assume liabilities.

In most cases, assets are purchased free from existing liabilities. For example, the seller includes inventory in the purchase price *without* transferring any accounts payable. The seller must settle these debts himself—which may be why he's asking for such a large down payment.

You can take advantage of this situation by assuming the liabilities and thus reduce the purchase price and the required down payment. You'll reap an additional benefit because you can then repay the debt from your practice cash flow over an extended period of time. You could also re-negotiate the loan balance on these assets to a larger amount.

Assuming liabilities can be a particularly effective strategy if the seller is willing to schedule his final accounts payable to come due as long after the closing date as possible.

4. Borrow from interested parties.

Banks loan money to earn interest income, but other institutions may be interested in loaning money in order to secure a valuable customer or commission. For example, if the seller has been leasing equipment or property, the leasing company may be willing to loan money to you, the buyer, to ensure that you'll continue the lease. Such arrangements are even more likely if the sale is being handled by the owner's estate, which may be considering closing the practice altogether.

You also may find a friend in a supplier salesperson who has made large commissions from the practice in the past. He or she might loan you money directly or agree to delay billing for supplies. A supplier interested in securing a new account may be willing to negotiate similar terms.

Another source is the practice broker, who will receive a large commission if the sale is completed. To avoid losing the sale, a practice broker may be willing to reduce his or her commission or loan you money from the commission—either of which could put you in a better position to close the sale.

5. Sublease excess facilities.

If there is excess space in the practice, consider subleasing. Tenants are easier to attract than you might imagine. Even in depressed economies, one-room offices usually remain in demand. And don't overlook parking areas, storage facilities or even equipment—all can be leased.

The best strategy is to find a tenant who will prepay all or part of the rent—thus providing you with part of the down payment on the practice's purchase price.

6. Lease-purchase.

Arranging a lease-purchase agreement is similar to asking the seller to finance the sale and usually means that he or she won't receive as much cash upon closing the deal. But the arrangement still can be attractive if it is structured so that the buyer retains tax benefits such as depreciation. A lease-purchase deal also can help the seller avoid having to recapture investment tax credit.

In addition, the seller may actually end up with more money from a lease-purchase arrangement because the financing costs are combined with a high final buy-out amount. And if the seller needs the cash at closing, he or she may be able to borrow against the lease agreements. Both the equipment and the lease have value as collateral, and the buyer's lease payments can be applied to the loan payments. The seller also could sell his or her equipment to a leasing company, lease it back and transfer the debt service to you.

7. Satisfy retirement needs.

Let's say the funds the seller receives from the sale of the practice will allow him or her to pay off any debt still owed on the practice. Then why would a large down payment still be needed? A practitioner looking forward to retirement may need that additional cash for a down payment on, say, a retirement home or recreational vehicle.

One way to meet both parties' needs is for the retiring doctor to finance his retirement purchase, and for you, the buyer, to service his debt. To reassure the seller, it's wise to arrange the loan for the shortest term possible.

8. Defer the down payment.

A seller who insists on a large down payment may lose in the long run because of an unfavorable tax position. That's why the tax implications may be enough to convince the seller to sweeten the deal. For example, a seller receiving a substantial portion of the sales price will pay taxes on any capital gains when the cash is received. If he or she practices up until the time of the sale, the seller will likely fall in a higher tax bracket, which means he or she will actually end up with less cash.

However, if a portion of the cash from the sale is deferred until the next tax year (or over several tax years), the seller's burden would be distributed over a time in which he or she likely would be in a lower tax bracket.

When you make the move to buy or sell a veterinary practice, remember that there are two sides to the sale and that both bring to it different objectives. The key to a successful negotiation is to openly discuss each party's needs, and then work together to meet them. Rather than relying solely on the purchase price negotiation, look for alternatives. The seller may be surprised to find that he or she can achieve desired results without insisting on a large amount of cash at closing.

Notes

Chapter 9:
Managing Miscellanies

Managing high technology

by Paul M. Schmitz, DVM, staff member of America Online's® Pet Care Forum's "Questions for Vets Area"

"Mom and Pop [have gone] high tech .... The little guys are rushing into the information age."

Computer Shopper magazine, December 1994

When I attended veterinary college in the late '70s and early '80s, computers were still rather large machines, used only by large companies. Now, however, computers have revolutionized corporations as well as home offices in the 1990s. Along with the home computing market, we have the "so-ho" (small office-home office) market as well. All of this is important to you as a veterinarian and hospital manager for a variety of reasons.

Quiet revolution

There is a quiet revolution in the way small companies view and use information technology. Embracing computer and network technology helps level the playing field for small businesses, including small veterinary hospitals versus the oncoming corporate giants in our profession.

State-of-the-art digital technology once available only to deep-pocketed companies or hospitals is making its way into "mom and pop" stores, clinics and homes. There's no turning back. The information has arrived on Main Street.

The forces that have reshaped Corporate America—greater competition, relentless cost-cutting and demands for higher quality—now reach businesses of every size in every segment of the economy, including solo veterinary practitioners.

State-of-the-art digital technology once available only to deep-pocketed companies or hospitals is making its way into "mom and pop" stores, clinics and homes. There's no turning back. The information has arrived on Main Street.

Megastores such as Wal-Mart, Home Depot, Office Max and PetsMart are forcing rival retailers, as well as merchandise suppliers and service providers, both small and large, to adopt sophisticated "high tech" equipment for record keeping, invoice generation, inventory management and electronic ordering. Along with this comes more use of computer-related technology for maintaining close contact not only with suppliers but with clients as well.

Digital revolution:*

Percent of US workers involved in information work: 55%
Industrial firm whose market value is less than Microsoft's:........................GM
Year sales of computers surpassed those of color televisions:..................1993
Year sales of encyclopedias on CD-ROM surpassed those on paper:.........1993
Percent of computers attached to networks in 1989: 10%
Percent of computers attached to networks in 1994: 60%
Percent of US homes that will have computers by end of 1994:..................30%
With answering machines:..40%
Number of people who work on computers in the home:..................40 million
Growth of traffic on the NSF backbone in one month (March 1994): 20.7%
Growth of World Wide Web traffic in same period: 32.9%
Percent of US homes with a child 8-12 with video games:............................70%
Gross US movie box office sales: ....$5 billion
Video game market in 1993:..$6 billion
CD-ROM players sold in 1989:..a few thousand
CD-ROM players sold in 1993: ....3.5 million
Market for interactive programming by 1998: ....$18.2 billion
Size of the US defense budget: ....$270 billion
Value of computer hardware and software sold in the US: ....$500 billion
·Estimated size of the telecommunications market in 2001: ....$1.3 trillion

* Source: *Wired Magazine,* Winter 1994-95

To computerize or not to computerize?

Many articles have been written on this subject, year after year, since the first veterinary hospitals began using personal computers. Ultimately, it is a personal decision, as well as a business decision, for every veterinarian. But be forewarned—if you are one of the "holdouts," don't wait too much longer.

As clients become more computer savvy, they will expect more from you as well. Remember, the next new client to walk through your door may be coming from a "high tech" hospital from some other city or state. This client will certainly be looking to see that you have a caring demeanor, superior medical skills and a clean hospital ... but he or she may also be looking to see if you're driving down the "information superhighway" as well.

If you haven't computerized yet (and I personally know of practices grossing $1 million or more at this writing that haven't) ... think again! In 1985, only 25 percent of small businesses reported having any computerization, and that percentage was probably high for our profession. By 1990, 67.5 percent were computerized ... still high for veterinary hospitals. Since 1992, the number of veterinary hospitals not yet computerized has continued to drop, year after year.

Being computerized, however, veterinarians and their staff are using less than 50 percent of their computers' capabilities to help them be more efficient, more thorough, more profitable veterinarians. I know of many hospitals that have been through two or more veterinary practice management systems to arrive at the level of practice computerization that they have today.

The greatest impediments to more extensive computer use have been a lack of resources and training ... until now, that is. The two biggest concerns practitioners have about adopting information technology are staff training and planning.

This may be changing. Hundreds of easy-to-use programs built on the Microsoft Windows® operating systems are now available.

And it's not just application programs ... small and large veterinary hospitals today can choose from easy-to-install computer networks, such as Novell Inc.'s NetWare® and Arti-Soft's Lantastic®. Networking capabilities never before available to so many users are offered by Windows for Workgroups® and the recently released Windows '95® (Chicago). Today's entrepreneurial success stories almost always include information technology.

Remember reminders?

Are you making full use of your computer for generating reminders? Does your veterinary system adequately track medical history, ancillary services and inventory the way you'd hoped it would? Does it perform detailed "criteria searches" to seek out those clients that fit a particular mold so you can generate more specific reminders, letters and newsletters?

If not, look around ... advances are still occurring in veterinary practice software. There may be another system out there for you. You may want to consider a graphical user interface (GUI) system instead of a DOS, UNIX or proprietary based system. Whether you are an "old pro" or just getting to the "on-ramp," you may find one of these new Windows®-based veterinary systems more to your or your staff's liking.

Computers as word processors

Initially, the first computers that we as veterinarians used were nothing more than primarily "reminder factories" with some "cash-registering" abilities and good billing abilities. Any word processing capabilities they had were limited at best. Unfortunately, this is still true for many veterinary systems which offer only "crudimentary" word processing integrated within the practice management system. The only real advantage of these systems are that they allow for smoother mail merge directly between documents and the client–patient database. Today, however, you can obtain some of the most sophisticated word processors "over-the-counter" for your desktop PC or Macintosh—whether "tower," desktop or laptop. The only difficulty, if there is one, is merging your custom letter or newsletter with your client–patient database. Continue to shop the veterinary system market, as improvements in this area continue to be made.

In my own experience, creating a separate database of client names and addresses is not that difficult—keeping them automatically current and updated, however, is (especially when it's outside your veterinary system)!

You can certainly produce excellent, professional-looking newsletters, letters, flyers, banners, client information handouts and even hospital forms by using these "friendlier programs;"

and now with computers at home or possibly a freestanding PC or Mac in the office, it is possible to have these kinds of programs readily available.

Get to know a good word processor or desktop publishing program. Some of the more popular ones include: WordPerfect® (DOS and Windows), MS Word for Windows®, Ami-Pro®, MS Publisher®, Ventura Publisher® and QuarkExpress® (Mac and Windows). Of course, all of these programs also accommodate graphics, which will always impress your clients and help your hospital grow.

Don't forget to use your computer for producing "real-time" information for your clients (e.g., feeding instructions via pet food programs like Hill's "Feeding Guide" and Purina's "CNM Feeding Guide & Nutritional Management Program"), client information sheets (e.g., Instructions for Veterinary Clients on diskette from Mosby) and your own custom-made instructional handouts. These can all be printed at patient discharge or client exit if your system is set up to allow for it ... and it should be!

Computers as diagnostic tools

Database sources: Veterinary computer software of the future will address the issues of medical history and retrieval via searchable databases built right into the veterinary practice management system.

As cases are worked up, the data or history from these cases will be added to an in-house database, which will eventually make it possible to do a search and come up with diagnostic "rule-outs" from your own data bank of cases and patients.

Presently, the only programs (and there are several to choose from) that do such computer-aided diagnostics are freestanding programs, such as Provides®; and the problem with this type of program is that it doesn't connect with the user's existing database very easily. Users therefore have been slow to really utilize the full features of such a program.

Time is also a factor in running such diagnostic programs. We need to learn to take the time to use this technology and charge for it … make it an income-generating service. Teach your technicians to use these programs too. Everyone will benefit if you do!

Reference sources: Presently, there are available several programs through which you can retrieve information about drugs and dosages (e.g., The Physicians' Desk Reference®, Plums Veterinary Drug Handbook, Target®, a new antimicrobial dosage calculating program, among many others). These references will prove to be very useful, and the selection will grow as time goes on.

You might want to also look at products like the Merck Veterinary Manual, Seventh Edition-Electronic Version on diskette —for DOS and Windows. Though many of us may not be turning to the Merck Manual in our daily practice lives, Merck has made fantastic strides at providing a complete book in an easy-to-read and searchable format that no hospital should be without.

Computers as communications tools

E-mail: Electronic mail (e-mail) is already making a big difference in the way we all communicate. Even for those of you afraid to jump onto the "superhighway," learning to use e-mail will at least help keep you from being run over. E-mail comes in all sorts of computer communications packages and is the foundation of many of the on-line computer services. Without e-mail, there would be little or no real communication occurring in "cyberspace." E-mail comes with its own language and etiquette (see the following sample of cyberspace shorthand) and usually is a faster method of communicating ideas to someone. It does, however, have some pitfalls; and you must bear this in mind when communicating in this medium.

Facial expression, body posture and voice intonation are not part of e-mail—so you must remember to always think first about what you say or write before you send it. Ask yourself, "Would I like to receive this letter?" "Flaming" (sending inflammatory mail) is common over some networks and bulletin board systems (BBS's) and should be avoided in professional situations (or at least among veterinarians.)

E-mail is not just a language of the big networks. It is available on almost every local area network (and some veterinary programs as well). Many of you will be using such a network in your hospital setting in the very near future, if you aren't already.

Privacy of e-mail is a concern; but depending on your system or network, it's not much of a problem. Just remember, if more than one person is using the system and you post public messages, everyone will see your messages — unless you stick to private e-mail only — with passwords.

Examples of cyberspace shorthand:

:) <—smiley face

:(<—sad face

;-) <—wink with nose and smile

:-o <—mouth open in surprise

<G> <—big grin

IMHO <—In My Humble Opinion

ROFLOL <—Rolling On Floor Laughing Out Loud

GMTA <—Great Minds Think Alike

BRB <—Be Right Back

Fax machines: Fax machines (which make facsimiles) are a critical component in today's business climate. Faxing enables your hospital to send and receive information quickly from your lab, suppliers, other veterinarians and specialists and even your clients (if not now, then in the future).

As more and more clients get fax machines of all kinds (today, virtually all computers go out with fax/modems installed), your ability to send out announcements, hospital catalogs, advertisements, newsletters or any important health information via fax will increase exponentially. Your clients will grow to expect this kind of high-speed information transfer. You should be asking clients (both old and new) for their fax numbers as part of your client information database.

There are fax/printer/copy machine combinations available for little more than the price of a basic laser printer. Some fax devices are built into scanning devices as well.

Fax machines continue to drop in price, print better and faster, and many use plain paper (like you'd use in your laser printer or copier). The lower-priced, freestanding fax machines (non-plain paper) run under $200. For even less money, you can invest in a fax/modem for your computer and receive faxes directly into your computer. The downside of this system is that any document you want to send must first be in your computer (on your hard drive or on a floppy disk).

Here's a trick for getting around the fax board dilemma on your computer when it comes to sending a fax: Try using your flatbed scanner (if you've invested in one) for scanning an image to your fax board. It works very well, although it takes a little practice and is a little more labor-intensive. A new feature in faxing is the "wireless" fax, which uses special fax modems and cellular phone technology. This is popular with laptop computer users, and pretty accurate.

Voice mail: Voice mail has been with us for some time. It started out as an answering machine and now has progressed to both on-site and off-site full-service, multiple-mailbox, computerized messaging centers. You can now have your own voice-mail system on your personal computer. Voice mail is more personal than a plain answering machine because it usually allows for unlimited length, more detailed messages from the caller. Having your friends, family members and ultimately clients use your voice mailbox is an easy way for them to leave you messages without disrupting the front personnel desk and tying up main phone lines unnecessarily. Just be sure and check in with your mailbox regularly, or callers will feel ignored or neglected pretty quickly—which can be more dangerous than having them not reach you at all. Most voice-mail systems can page you remotely to let you know you have a voice-mail message.

On-hold messages: Another popular promotional tool is the "on-hold" phone message. Most of us hate silence when we are put on hold. With or without sophisticated phone equipment, just about everyone can afford to have customized on-hold messages. Many companies are offering such services at reasonable rates and with regular updates.

It's actually pretty easy to do these yourself (with a little ingenuity), and your clients might enjoy listening to their doctor's voice while waiting to make an appointment to see you "in the flesh."

Cellular phones: Cellular technology is rapidly advancing to where now a large segment of your clients probably have cellular phones at their disposal. The use of a cellular phone in your practice can replace the pager (at a price), but I would recommend you have the client use that phone number for emergency calls only—rates haven't gotten that low yet, and you usually pay for all time spent on the cellular network, whether you placed the call or not.

The day may come when charges are more balanced; but even now, having that phone with you can come in handy when you really need it. I know of some practices in remodeling situations and during catastrophic emergencies (hurricanes or earthquakes) that made use of cellular phones to such a degree that the phones were literally lifelines to the outside world and their client base— and without them, these practices might have perished.

Pet tip hotlines: Pet tip hotlines are becoming increasingly popular. Some are national 800 numbers; some are 900 numbers that are used to raise money for certain causes (e.g., shelters, humane societies); and some are simply local numbers that clients can call to hear recorded pet health tips and learn more about your practice. To have such a hotline, you must usually invest in a computerized voice-mail system and a dedicated phone line; but you may find companies in your area (e.g., the yellow pages) that are offering limited service, similar but smaller in scope, for an additional monthly fee along with your yellow pages bill.

The purpose of such a venture should not be completely altruistic in nature. It should attract new clients and educate existing ones about your hospital services and products. A pet tip hotline is another example of keeping your hospital's name in front of your clients and potential clients. For people to call, you must promote such a service. Remember, though, many people will not call such a service; and those that do will certainly not listen for more than a couple of minutes at a time per tip. Make your messages short (under two to three minutes, tops; but they can be longer than your on-hold messages), promote them heavily as public service messages and try to regularly track the number of callers.

You can stay ahead of your colleagues by instituting a help line. It's not likely they will do the same thing ... at least not right away. Be the first one on your block ... and then work on being the best at offering a pet tip hotline later! For several examples of actual hotline tips, see the accompanying *Practice Workbook*, Section 11: Marketing Protocols—Part One.

Electronic bulletin board systems (BBS's): An on-line computer bulletin board for your hospital? For your clients? Electronic bulletin board systems may be the wave of the future! You should be looking at this as an exciting new opportunity to reach hundreds, possibly thousands, of new clients. An electronic

BBS is a computer community or forum, much like the larger networks (e.g., America Online®, CompuServe® and Prodigy®), but usually much smaller in scope. I once heard it said that a BBS is like the local station affiliate when compared to the big networks of the television industry.

It takes some skill, and possibly a more advanced interest in computers and BBS's to be the sysop (systems operator) and designer of such a service; but given the number of potential customers that eventually can be reached this way, it may be worth the effort. A BBS can be labor-intensive at first, if started from the ground up; but with some planning and some research, you can find the system that will work best for your needs. Many systems are very easy to use and could probably be maintained by a staff person, perhaps a technician or an interested associate veterinarian.

Some experienced veterinarians you know have probably explored this exciting new area and may be able to offer you assistance in setting up your own hospital BBS. I have recently set one up for the Woodland PetCare Centers group of practices here in Tulsa.

Through a BBS, your hospital will be able to communicate to a whole new group of people ... many of whom are highly articulate and may be just the type of client you've been hoping to attract to your hospital. Of course, there are those that just "hang out" on the BBS, playing games, causing chaos and simply chatting with others on-line. These may not all make suitable clients, but at least they may become more exposed to veterinary medicine by being a part of your electronic community.

A BBS that is set up properly, one that has quality pet health information and fun facts about pets, is sure to get attention among BBS browsers. You can include all sorts of pet health information for pet-owning users to read and download, such as pictures or examples of disease conditions to download. You also have the ability to carry on chats and send e-mail to other friends and pet lovers on-line.

If you become the first to offer a BBS, your hospital can become the "talk of the town." Be aware, though, that this initially may not be a money-making venture. It is mostly a public relations enterprise, for now; but it is public (client) education at its best! The ability to generate an income from your BBS will come later as new clients are exposed to your forward thinking in putting free pet information on-line for them. There are ways to make your BBS actually produce income by charging people for downloading of valuable information. Programs are readily available that allow you to charge to a person's credit card and then credit your account, automatically. There are many excellent publications about BBS's available from your local book store or library.

On-line services: America Online®, CompuServe®, Prodigy®, Delphi®, Genie® and the Internet are all on-line computer services or networks. Some are bigger than others, and some are catering to the needs and interests of veterinarians more than others.

With the explosion of veterinary medical knowledge, it is extremely difficult for most veterinarians to stay current. Many states have continuing education (CE) requirements for veterinarians. Obtaining CE is difficult to do with the rigors of practice. Information is increasing at the rate of over 35 percent per year with over 6,000 new scientific articles per day. Let's assume that only one percent of these impact on the practice of veterinary medicine. This would mean that even if you read one new article a day, by the end of the year, you would be behind the pace of keeping "totally up" by over 50 years! Computer communications promise to make this problem much less significant.

These on-line services change every hour of every day. It is whatever the veterinarians on-line that particular day want it to be. Some days it is a source of the latest information, *months and years ahead* of the printed journals. Other days it is a place to exchange e-mail messages with other veterinarians. The essense of these networks is their ability to conform to the needs of their members while maintaining a strong sense of community.

The Veterinary Information Network (VIN), on America Online®, and the AVMA's Network of Animal Health (NOAH), on CompuServe®, are both addressing the overwhelming problem of managing veterinary information. VIN was the first computer-based information network available to practicing veterinarians in this country. Either service gives any veterinarian with a computer and access to America Online® or CompuServe® the ability to communicate with thousands of veterinarians nationwide on a daily basis. This communication takes place between both those in private practice and those at the university level.

The Internet is a world of its own and will become another one of the meeting places of the future. Access to this "network of networks" opens up innumerable possibilities. By joining various Internet "mailing lists," you can also participate in personalized, in-depth electronic discussions about numerous veterinary topics. Some of the available groups are as follows: Veterinary Informatics, Veterinary Hospital Information and general veterinary medicine mailing lists.

In many ways, on-line services are like libraries dedicated to the veterinary profession, with summaries of several years of veterinary publications and postings by practitioners and academicians alike. In fact, an on-line service is one of the few meeting places where practitioners and academicians cross paths on a daily basis. This benefits everyone in the profession. Imagine how useful it would be for you to be able to almost immediately communicate with board-certified specialists and fellow practitioners with similar experiences on a problem case.

Literature retrieval is already one of the primary uses of any of these networks and will become more valuable as more journals (scientific and nonscientific) go on-line. The National Library of Medicine (NLM) maintains one of the largest literature retrieval services that can be accessed through software such as Grateful Med. Since the NLM service is a government-supported service, the cost of being on-line is minimal; but as of yet, this service does little to truly cover veterinary medicine, as it is mostly a human medicine database-retrieval service.

Interactive video conferencing: Face-to-face meetings with colleagues are now possible for most veterinarians that are traveling "up to speed" on the "information highway"—all without traveling more than an hour from their homes or offices to a video-conferencing center.

Transmitting documents, radiographs, echocardiograms, ultrasounds and entire books in a matter of minutes is already possible; but being able to have real-time video imaging to meet with people "face to face" without having to travel will soon be a great new option for us all.

On-line "rounds" sessions in computer forums like VIN will more than likely soon be combined with real-time video—it's just a matter of time before we catch up with technology. It is the next frontier of the information age.

You will also see such services as America Online® moving towards interactive television with their computer network, probably within the next one to two years.

Toys to business tools

Some of the many "high-tech toys" now available for you to use in your business include the following:

- Laptop computers;

- PDAs (personal digital assistants);

- Digital cameras (for taking digital photographs of interesting cases or patients);

- Voice command software so your computer can respond to your spoken voice (I see this coming for veterinary systems at the front desk.);

- Handheld and flatbed scanners; and

- Digital TV and radio for client-oriented educational programs or for professional continuing education.

Conclusion

Total information is doubling every three years and is likely to change even faster as we near the new millennium. This chapter was very difficult to write because of the ever-changing nature of its contents. There is sure to be new technology on the market by the time this book is published and you have had the time to buy it and read it all the way to this chapter. To not take full advantage of today's and tomorrow's technology is to follow a formula for financial failure as well as failure to deliver the best quality of medicine available.

In-house lab equipment vs. professional lab services

by David B. Goodnight, DVM, MBA, practitioner in Dallas, Tex.

Many veterinarians purchase in-house lab equipment in an attempt to offer more and better service to their clients. That's no surprise, considering the recent advances in technology and the need to remain competitive in today's environment. The equipment now available makes it possible for veterinarians to provide testing with immediate feedback and a high degree of accuracy.

Many clinics now offer routine presurgical chemistry screens, a service not previously performed by some because of the logistical and timing problems associated with sending blood to a commercial lab. In addition, an in-house lab also allows veterinarians to perform follow-up testing on animals under treatment and to quickly verify or rule out diagnostic suspicions, all of which can potentially enhance client satisfaction. Immediate feedback also gives the clinician the opportunity to complete the exam and diagnostic process in one visit, avoiding costly, uncompensated phone conversations at a later time. Technology is moving so rapidly with the addition of new tests not previously possible in-house that in many cases in-house lab equipment can now replace the routine use of commercial labs.

Purchasing such equipment can offer some real advantages, but attention must always be paid to the business aspect of any decision to buy. The practitioner must make sure that the service offered by that equipment yields adequate profit to justify the purchase economically. Veterinarians should not deal from emotion or the perceived pressures of professional competitiveness (i.e., what everyone else is doing). Purchasing decisions must be made at the business level. They merit some analysis or capital budgeting to determine the acquisition's economic viability.

Large companies use techniques such as net present value calculations (NPV), internal rate of return (IRR) or payback.

These are valid approaches, but in my opinion they lack practicality for use in most small veterinary clinics. Small businesses should use simple analysis methods with immediate and ongoing applicability, particularly when the equipment generates measurable income streams on a stand-alone basis.

Before making any purchase, it is smart to make some realistic projections for use. Historical surgical and medical loads will help predict future use for presurgical screenings and day-to-day use in medical cases, respectively. Estimates must also be made to predict how much lab work will be shifted from commercial labs to in-house. A more difficult projection to make is how many additional lab tests you will perform once the equipment is readily accessible.

Even after purchasing it, you should monitor the equipment's use to make sure it is performing to your level of expectation and contributing to profit in a significant manner.

When lab equipment is being sold to practices, vendors of lab equipment often try to demonstrate how few tests actually have to be run to "pay for the equipment." This is a seriously flawed calculation. Although everyone should be interested in paying for the equipment, they should be more interested in the profit it will generate above that point. You can *always* make a profit by sending work to a commercial lab. Most of us have that option already—even if we don't utilize it as much as we should.

Buyers beware

Vendors also try to convince you that you will "run more lab tests" if you have in-house equipment available. This may be true in theory, but not in reality. To buy based on the assumption that your lab volume will increase (and in some cases *must* increase to make economic sense) is risky. This is an individual decision each veterinarian must make.

With the purchase of in-house lab equipment, commitment to sustained use is essential because it creates fixed overhead (a payment or an investment opportunity lost) for the practice—whether you use the equipment or not. You do not have fixed overhead using commercial labs, only incremental costs (the cost of the profile, syringe, etc.).

Vendors also tend to present returns in terms of total dollars earned instead of accounting returns to the practice. Don't just accept this information at face value. Make sure the equipment performs to your profit expectations. One vendor once tried to give an income comparison of the same test in-house and at a commercial lab, ignoring the fixed costs of owning the equipment and addressing only the variable costs (reagents). When pressed about the exclusion, the explanation was, "Well, you are investing in equipment that will give value to your practice; whereas, sending lab work out to a commercial lab does nothing for the value of your practice." We found that answer nonresponsive.

After further discussion, the vendor explained that "all you have to do is average the fixed costs over the monthly tests and add it to the price and pass it on to the client." He said the client would "never know because this is not a service that is shopped." Our interpretation: *It costs more to perform tests in-house.*

The point is: Identify all of the costs of owning and performing in-house lab tests and compare them with what you are currently doing so that you can make intelligent decisions. Don't be talked into buying without first evaluating whether it makes good business sense for your practice.

Premises of the analysis

I believe that if you purchase any piece of equipment, the service generated by that equipment should generate profit *and* produce a predetermined minimal return to the hospital. In-house lab equipment is not an exception. To evaluate profitability, I compare in-house testing to the same or comparable services offered with reasonable turnaround time by commercial labs. In-house lab revenues should return, at a minimum, the same percentage of gross profit you could earn from sending your lab work out to a commercial lab, even if the service is an additional service not previously offered.

I chose the word "minimum" because ownership allows for immediate results, allowing better service and care when it is necessary, and probably deserves a premium return over outside labs. Also, some or all of the lab work that would have been sent out will be replaced by in-house testing, and any potential profit should at least be equal or you would be harming yourself financially. This gives a working definition of what I referred to earlier as an "adequate profit."

Data presentation

The following abbreviated income statements (Figure 1A) demonstrate how the numbers were determined for the graphs and pricing matrices. With an in-house lab, the costs are composed of fixed (monthly payments) and variable (reagents, maintenance, syringes, etc.) expenses; whereas, sending lab work out is purely a variable expense (incremental profile cost, syringes, etc.). Gross profit and gross profit percentage are the two references used for profitability.

Gross profit is defined here as the total income for tests minus the reagent costs (or outside lab fee) minus the equipment payment. Gross profit percentage is derived by dividing the gross profit by the total income from the tests.

The graphs used throughout this analysis are designed to demonstrate the relationship between average price and the number of tests performed, both in-house and at a commercial lab, presented as the break-even point of gross profits.

The break-even point is defined as the point at which the same number of tests performed in-house or commercially would produce equal gross profit in total dollars. This break-even point can be important when deciding if you have adequate volume to justify a purchase.

In addition, I have included portions of the relative pricing matrices, using a data table analysis to change two variables, tests performed and average price per test to show their relationship to gross profit as a percentage. The matrix may seem like a complex way to evaluate a simple percentage return on gross revenue calculation, but I wanted to show the effects of volume against average pricing in a concise manner and offer a quick method of reference for performance. The pricing matrix offers a quick reference to adjust your price or volume, if possible, to achieve desired and necessary returns.

General assumptions

For ease in this study, it is assumed that the equipment is leased for a three-year period and that the payments used are from actual lease contracts currently in effect or from estimated quotes from vendors. The same analysis could be performed on a purchase basis using interest and depreciation as expenses in place of lease payments. Gross profit was used as a reference to avoid having to allocate any fixed costs of administrative overhead, since it is our opinion that it would not significantly change with in-house testing or the use of a commercial lab. Additional costs associated with training and the operation of in-house equipment were not quantified for this comparison since ease of operation is common with today's products and it is doubtful that labor would increase or decrease.

The analysis also does not consider any increased profits realized after the lease period because it is reasonable to expect that, with today's technology, the equipment will be obsolete in three years and could be returned or replaced with newer technology.

The average reagent cost for the chemistry analyzer in this analysis was $2.36 and the reagent cost for the cell counter was $2.75 per test performed. The fixed monthly payment for the cell counter is $354.00, and the fixed monthly payment for the chemistry analyzer is $243.62. Your assumptions may vary from the ones used, but anyone with any minor accounting experience can modify this analysis to their own situation with little effort.

Cell-counter comparison

It is easiest to use a single piece of test equipment, such as a cell counter, to compare in-house testing with outside testing. In our experience, a cell counter is the piece of equipment that is most likely to be used in place of outside testing.

The numbers used are actual fees from a national lab and a commonly used cell counter. Traditionally, if a CBC sent to an outside lab costs $9.00, most veterinarians charge the client $18.00, or a 100-percent markup with a 50-percent gross profit margin. As a starting point, the price charged the client for in-house testing was the same as the outside lab, in this case $18.00, the rationale being that it would seem logical to charge a client the same fee for the same service–unless you believe that immediate feedback deserves a premium; and if you use that argument, you must determine how much of a premium is justified and adjust the calculations accordingly.

The graph in Figure 1A and income statement in Figure 1B show the break-even point for in-house CBCs versus use of a commercial lab.

It appears that with prices being equal at $18.00, you would have to perform approximately 57 CBCs per month in-house before it would become more profitable than sending them to an outside lab. Another way to look at the same thing is to look at the pricing matrix in Figure 1C.

Income Statement

Figure 1A

Tests Per Month In-House CBC **$18.00 Per Test**	13	20	27	34	41	48	57
Total Revenue Per Month	$234	$360	$486	$612	$738	$864	$1,026
Variable Expense Per Month	$36	$55	$74	$94	$113	$132	$157
Fixed Cost Per Month	$354	$354	$354	$354	$354	$354	$354
Gross Profit Per Month	($156)	($49)	$58	$165	$271	$378	$515
Gross Profit %	−67%	−14%	12%	27%	37%	44%	50%
Tests Per Month Outside Lab CBC **$18.00 Per Test**	13	20	27	34	41	48	57
Total Revenue Per Month	$234	$360	$486	$612	$738	$864	$1,026
Variable Expense Per Month	$117	$180	$243	$306	$369	$432	$515
Fixed Cost Per Month	$0.00	$0.00	$0.00	$0.00	$0.00	$0.00	$0.00
Gross Profit Per Month	$117	$180	$243	$306	$369	$432	$513
Gross Profit %	50%	50%	50%	50%	50%	50%	50%

CBC Gross Profits

IN-HOUSE VS. COMMERCIAL

Figure 1B

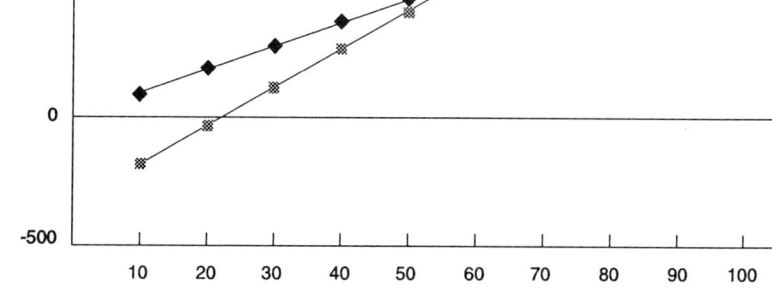

$ 18.00 Per Test in-House or Commercial

Pricing Matrix For In-House CBC Units Vs. Average Price Per Test

GROSS PROFIT MARGIN

TESTS PERFORMED ->

	13	20	27	34	41	48	57	64	71
$ 18.00	−67%	−14%	12%	27%	37%	44%	50%	54%	57%
$ 18.50	−62%	−11%	14%	29%	38%	45%	52%	55%	58%
$ 19.00	−58%	−8%	17%	31%	40%	47%	53%	56%	59%
$ 19.50	−54%	−5%	19%	33%	42%	48%	54%	58%	60%
$ 20.00	−50%	−2%	21%	34%	43%	49%	55%	59%	61%
$ 20.50	−46%	0%	23%	36%	44%	51%	56%	60%	62%
$ 21.00	−43%	3%	24%	37%	46%	52%	57%	61%	63%

It is easy to pick a price and number of tests and quickly see the return represented as a gross profit percentage. With price being the same, the 50-percent box on the pricing matrix represents the point at which the lines cross on the graph. This is not so if the prices are different, as you will observe in the next example. Approximately 57 CBCs yield a percentage gross profit of 50 percent. Look at the discrepancy in gross profits at smaller volumes, 20 and 27 units, when priced the same.

If you run fewer tests than 57, you will have to charge more per in-house test than outside lab test to realize the same profit. For example, if you are historically only running 34 tests per month, you must charge $26.50 per in-house test to achieve the same gross profit percentage (see Figure 2C) you would make by sending the tests outside at $18.00.

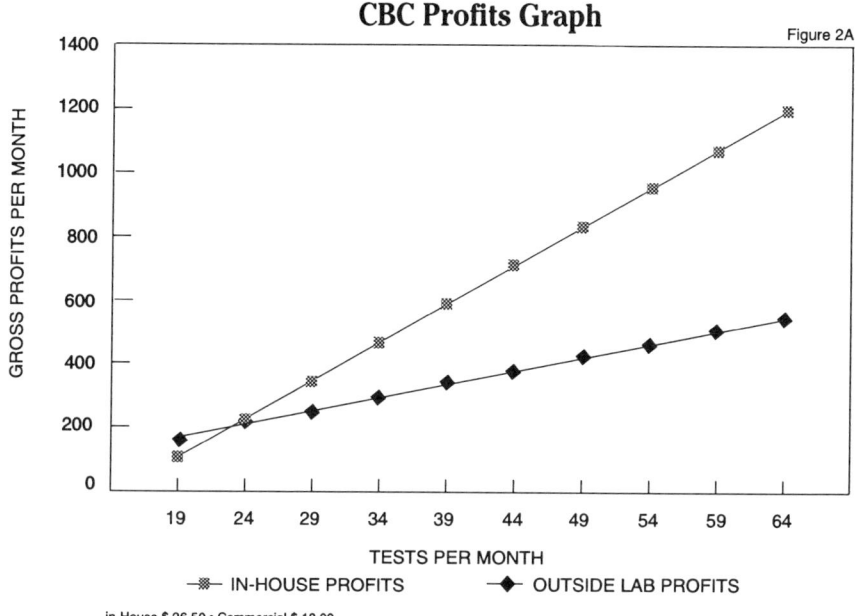

CBC Profits Graph

Figure 2A

in-House $ 26.50 • Commercial $ 18.00

The graph in Figure 2A can be a little misleading when the pricing of the tests is different. In this case, the in-house CBC is $26.50 and the commercial CBC is $18.00. The graph gives the impression that in-house testing becomes more profitable after the 24th test. This is true in terms of total gross profit dollars, but the gross profit percentage is only 34 percent in-house versus 50 percent with the commercial lab because you must gross more total dollars in-house than with the outside lab to earn the same gross profit dollars. Figure 2B demonstrates that it takes $636.00 gross revenue in-house versus $432.00 gross revenue with the outside lab to earn the same $216.00 of gross profit. If you require a 50-percent gross profit percentage, you must gross $901.00 in-house before you achieve your goal (Figure 2B).

Income Statement

Figure 2B

Tests Per Month In-House CBC	19	24	29	34	39	44
$26.50 Per Test						
Total Revenue Per Month	$504	$636	$769	$901	$1,034	$1,166
Variable Expense Per Month	$52	$66	$80	$94	$107	$121
Fixed Cost Per Month	$354	$354	$354	$354	$354	$354
Gross Profit Per Month	$97	$216	$335	$454	$572	$691
Gross Profit %	19%	34%	44%	50%	55%	59%
Tests Per Month Outside Lab CBC	19	24	29	34	39	44
$18.00 Per Test						
Total Revenue Per Month	$342	$432	$522	$612	$702	$792
Variable Expense Per Month	$171	$216	$261	$306	$351	$396
Fixed Cost Per Month	$0.00	$0.00	$0.00	$0.00	$0.00	$0.00
Gross Profit Per Month	$171	$216	$261	$306	$351	$396
Gross Profit %	50%	50%	50%	50%	50%	50%

Figure 2C

Pricing Matrix For In-House CBC Units Vs. Average Price Per Test

GROSS PROFIT MARGIN

TESTS PERFORMED ->

	19	24	29	34	39	44	49	54
$ 25.00	14%	30%	40%	47%	53%	57%	60%	63%
$ 25.50	16%	31%	41%	48%	54%	58%	61%	64%
$ 26.00	18%	33%	42%	49%	55%	58%	62%	64%
$ 26.50	19%	34%	44%	50%	55%	59%	62%	65%
$ 27.00	21%	35%	45%	51%	56%	60%	63%	66%
$ 27.50	22%	36%	46%	52%	57%	61%	64%	66%
$ 28.00	24%	38%	47%	53%	58%	61%	64%	67%
$ 28.50	25%	39%	48%	54%	59%	62%	65%	67%
$ 29.00	26%	40%	48%	55%	59%	63%	66%	68%

Chemistry analyzer comparison

The cell-counter comparison was much more simple than the chemistry-analyzer comparison. The chemistry analyzer offers a variety of services, single tests through 10 to 12 test profiles. The average charge per test is lower in a profile than when performed individually, making a simple analysis difficult.

The most efficient way to monitor the results of the chemistry analyzer is to use the average charge per test received as a reference point. This allows for a combination of single tests performed blended with profiles that may be quantity discounted. Just track the total number of tests performed along with the total revenue generated and determine the average charge per test for analysis. The pricing matrix allows you to quickly reference the total number of individual tests performed and choose an average price to achieve your desired gross profit percentage.

For the purpose of analysis only, Figure 3A demonstrates a comparison of single tests performed in-house to those performed in a commercial lab using the same rationale as used for the cell counter.

On single chemistries, a national lab charges $6.00 per test. Following the same logic as presented above, a typical veterinarian would charge for the test. Figure 3A demonstrates the break-even point, as defined above, for running these tests on in-house equipment.

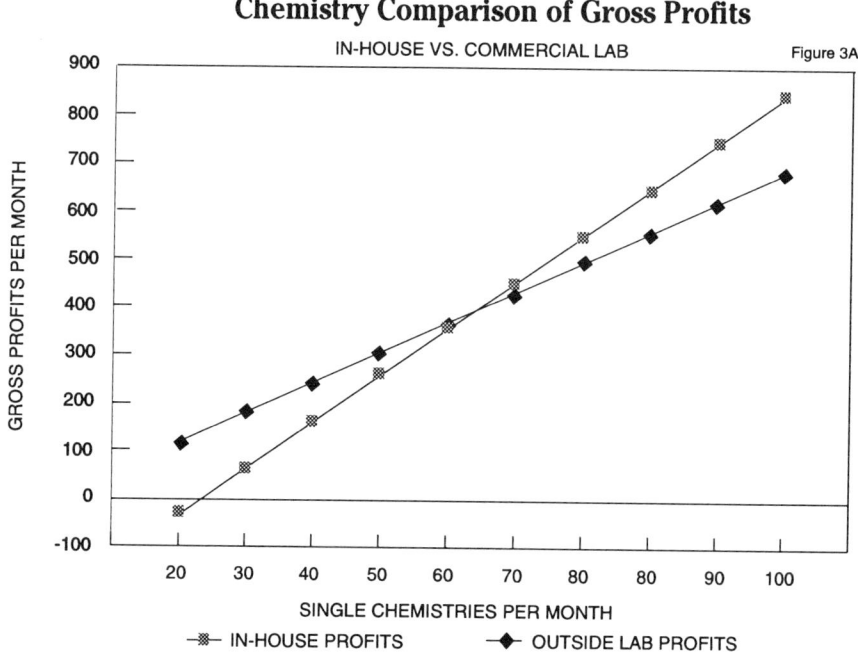

Chemistry Comparison of Gross Profits

IN-HOUSE VS. COMMERCIAL LAB

Figure 3A

Average Revenue - $ 12.00 Per Test Performed

Income Statement

Figure 3B

	20	30	62	68	74
Tests Per Month In-House Chemistry					
Average $12.00 Per Test					
Total Revenue Per Month	$240	$360	$744	$816	$888
Variable Expense Per Month	$47	$71	$146	$160	$175
Fixed Cost Per Month	$243.62	$243.62	$243.62	$243.62	$243.62
Gross Profit Per Month	$(51)	$46	$354	$412	$470
Gross Profit %	−21%	12%	48%	50%	53%
Tests Per Month Outside Lab Chemistry	20	30	62	68	74
Average $12.00 Per Test					
Total Revenue Per Month	$240	$360	$744	$816	$888
Variable Expense Per Month	$120	$180	$372	$408	$444
Fixed Cost Per Month	$0.00	$0.00	$0.00	$0.00	$0.00
Gross Profit Per Month	$120	$180	$372	$408	$444
Gross Profit %	50%	50%	50%	50%	50%

A glance at Figure 3B shows that *approximately 68 single tests a month at $6.00 per test are needed before it becomes more profitable to test in-house.*

For mini-profiles, a national lab charges $11.00 for six tests. *If you followed the same logic and charged $22.00 for the same six tests in-house, you could never perform enough profiles to make more profit in-house* because the variable costs of the tests are approximately $2.36 per test (Figures 4A & 4B).

Chemistry Comparison of Gross Profits

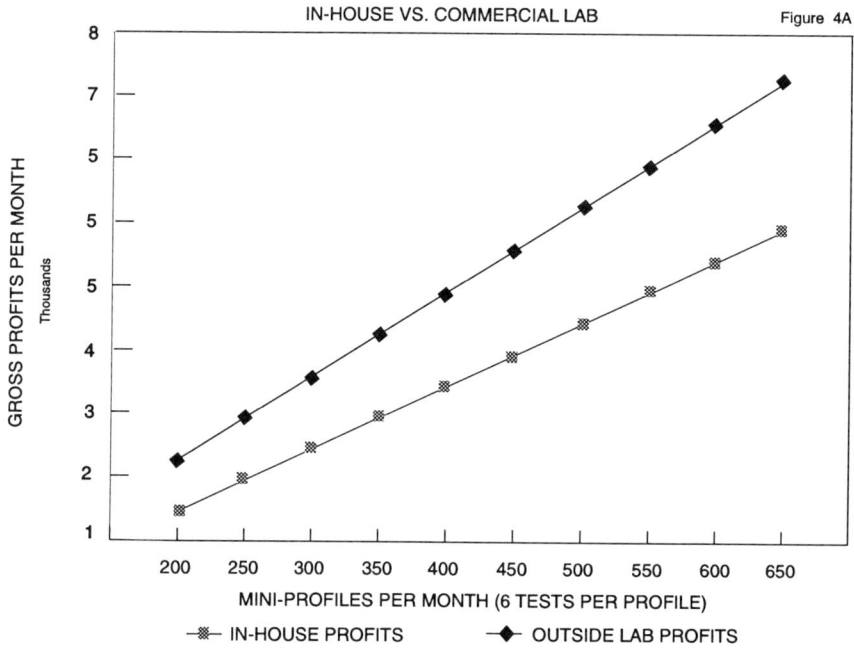

IN-HOUSE VS. COMMERCIAL LAB   Figure 4A

MINI-PROFILES PER MONTH (6 TESTS PER PROFILE)

—※— IN-HOUSE PROFITS   —◆— OUTSIDE LAB PROFITS

Revenue Pesr Test $ 22.00 In-House • $ 22.00 Outside Lab

Income Statement

Figure 4B

In-House Chemistry

Cost Per Mini-Profile (6 Tests)	$14.16			
Cost Per Test	$2.36			
Average Revenue Per Mini-Profile	$22.00			
Average Revenue Per Test	$3.67			
Tests Per Month In-House		200	250	300
Total Revenue Per Month		$4,400	$5,500	$6,600
Variable Expense Per Month		$2,832	$3,540	$4,248
Fixed Cost Per Month		$243.62	$243.62	$243.62
Gross Profit Per Month		$1,324	$1,716	$2,108
Gross Profit %		30%	31%	32%

Commercial Chemistry

Cost Per Mini-Profile (6 Tests)	$11.00			
Revenue Per Mini-Profile	$22.00			
Cost Per Test	$1.83			
Tests Per Month Outside Lab		200	250	300
Total Revenue Per Month		$4,400	$5,500	$6,600
Variable Expense Per Month		$2,200	$2,750	$3,300
Fixed Cost Per Month		$0.00	$0.00	$0.00
Gross Profit Per Month		$2,200	$2,750	$3,300
Gross Profit %		50%	50%	50%

Looking at the graph in Figure 5A, if you charged $35.00 to a client for the same six tests you could have performed at a commercial lab for a charge of $22.00, it appears to require only 23 profiles before it is more profitable in-house.

Chemistry Comparison of Gross Profits

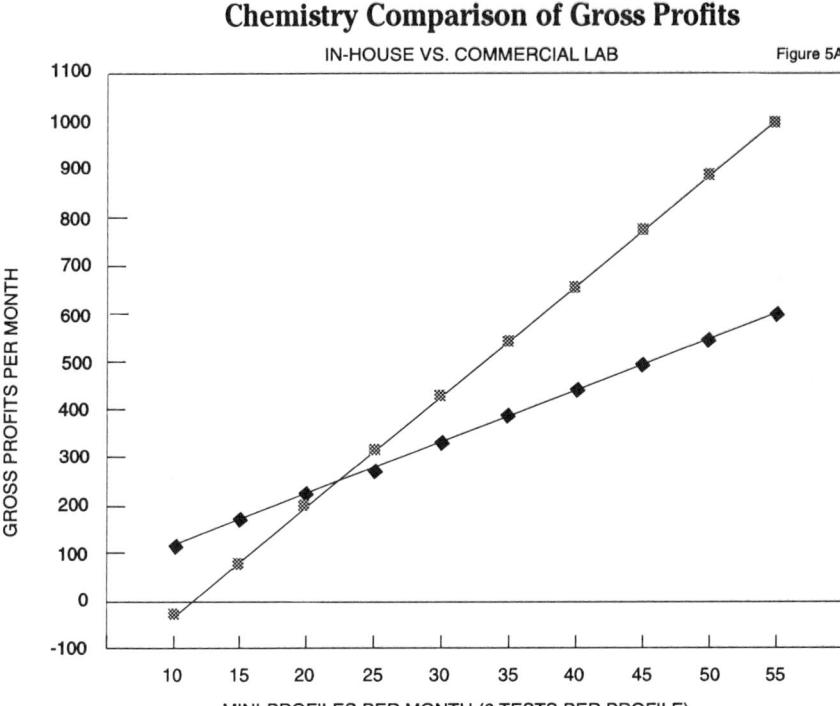

IN-HOUSE VS. COMMERCIAL LAB   Figure 5A

MINI-PROFILES PER MONTH (6 TESTS PER PROFILE)

—※— IN-HOUSE PROFITS   —◆— OUTSIDE LAB PROFITS

Revenue Per Test $ 35.00 In-House • $ 22.00 Outside Lab

Again, this is total dollars returned (Figures 5B and 5C). The percentage return is only 29 percent. At 23 profiles you would still have to gross $805.00 with the in-house equipment–as compared to $506.00 with a commercial lab–to end up with fewer gross profit dollars in-house. Does it make good "business sense" to have to gross that much more to earn less gross profit? If you want a 40-percent gross profit return, you would have to perform approximately 37 profiles per month charging the same $35.00; and if you want a 50-percent return, you would have to perform just over 65 profiles per month to achieve that return charging the higher price. This clearly demonstrates what the vendor was explaining in the introduction when discussing the need to spread fixed costs over each profile and pass it on to the client.

Income Statement

Figure 5B

Tests Per Month In-House Mini-Profile	9	16	23	30	65
Average $ 35.00 Per Profile					
Total Revenue Per Month	$315	$560	$805	$1,050	$2,275
Variable Expense Per Month	$127	$227	$326	$425	$920
Fixed Cost Per Month	$243.62	$243.62	$243.62	$243.62	$243.62
Gross Profit Per Month	$(56)	$90	$236	$382	$1,111
Gross Profit %	−18%	16%	29%	36%	49%
Tests Per Month Outside Lab Mini-Profile	9	16	23	30	65
Average $ 22.00 Per Profile					
Total Revenue Per Month	$198	$352	$506	$660	$1,430
Variable Expense Per Month	$99	$176	$253	$330	$715
Fixed Cost Per Month	$0.00	$0.00	$0.00	$0.00	$0.00
Gross Profit Per Month	$99	$176	$253	$330	$715
Gross Profit %	50%	50%	50%	50%	50%

Figure 5C

Pricing Matrix For In-House CBC Units Vs. Average Price Per Test

GROSS PROFIT MARGIN

MINI-PROFILES PERFORMED (6 TESTS PER MINI-PROFILE)

	19	16	23	30	37	44	65
$ 33.00	−25%	11%	25%	32%	37%	40%	46%
$ 34.00	−21%	14%	27%	34%	39%	42%	47%
$ 35.00	−18%	16%	29%	36%	41%	44%	49%
$ 36.00	−15%	18%	31%	38%	42%	45%	50%
$ 37.00	−11%	21%	33%	40%	44%	47%	52%
$ 38.00	−8%	23%	35%	41%	45%	48%	53%
$ 39.00	−6%	25%	37%	43%	47%	49%	54%
$ 40.00	−3%	27%	38%	44%	48%	51%	55%

Except for the value of immediate feedback and additional services not previously possible, it appears that the better economic value for the client and hospital can usually be achieved by having an outside lab perform multiple tests. If you own the equipment, you are obligated to make it profitable. Again, the intangible benefits (immediate feedback, phone-time conservation, etc.) are not quantified.

How to use this information

On a recent evaluation of a clinic with a chemistry analyzer, my associates and I took the total number of tests performed and total revenue generated over the previous nine months and determined an average charge per test and the average number of tests performed per month. Using computer data available, we further determined that this clinic was performing about 10 percent of the volume on individual tests and 90 percent on multiple tests.

The total revenue for the previous nine months was $8,199.00 and the total number of tests performed was 1,594. This calculates out to an average of $5.14 per test on 177 tests per month.

A quick look at the pricing matrix (Figure 5D) shows that the return to the clinic was approximately 25 percent.

Figure 5D

Pricing Matrix For In-House Chemistry Units

GROSS PROFIT MARGIN

TESTS PERFORMED ->

	50	75	100	125	150	175	200
$ 4.50	−61%	−25%	−7%	4%	11%	17%	20%
$ 5.00	−45%	−12%	4%	14%	20%	25%	28%
$ 5.50	−31%	−2%	13%	22%	28%	32%	35%
$ 6.00	−21%	7%	20%	28%	34%	37%	40%
$ 6.50	−11%	14%	26%	34%	39%	42%	45%
$ 7.00	−3%	20%	31%	38%	43%	46%	49%
$ 7.50	4%	25%	36%	43%	47%	50%	52%
$ 8.00	10%	30%	40%	46%	50%	53%	55%
$ 8.50	15%	34%	44%	49%	53%	56%	58%
$ 9.00	20%	38%	47%	52%	56%	58%	60%
$ 9.50	24%	41%	50%	55%	58%	61%	62%

Since we recommend a minimal 50-percent return, we suggested an average price of $7.50 at this volume. Now, to achieve the average, we offer two methods: First, charge for each and every test a fee of $7.50, whether you perform a single test or five tests. Second, use weighted average to determine the price per test.

Example:

Ninety percent of the tests were in multiple-test profiles and 10 percent of the tests were single tests. The first test of each multiple-test profile was considered a single test.

Equation : $(.90 \ A) + (.10 \ B) = 7.50$
(A = # multiple tests; B = # single tests)

Of course this equation can be solved with many different combinations of A and B. Therefore, we suggest that a fee be established for a single test, and the equation solved to determine A. For instance, if you decide you must have a minimum of $15.00 for a single test, solving the equation gives a price of $6.67 for each subsequent test. We suggest rounding to $6.75 to compensate for calibration and lost reagent costs.

Using the same matrix, if the same clinic had an average of 150 tests a month, you can quickly see that an average charge per test of $8.00 would be necessary to achieve the desired 50-percent return. Solving the equation above for the $8.00 average gives you a price of $15.00 for the first test and $7.22 (rounded to $7.25) for each multiple test sequence.

This is an easy technique to apply in your own office on a monthly or quarterly basis. You must continually monitor the results you are getting and be careful not to overcharge. If you examine all of your costs, track the number of tests performed, track the ratio of single tests to multiple tests and create a simple matrix, you can establish your desired return on gross profit and easily keep your equipment within profit compliance.

Summary

Cost-structure differences necessitate making in-house test fees higher than commercial lab fees with relative markup in order to reach the same gross profit level in total dollars and especially to achieve equality in gross profit percentage. The examples demonstrate that the fixed costs of ownership make it more difficult to realize the profits you can achieve with an outside lab, particularly at lower volumes.

Even if you argue that these are services you didn't offer before, you still have to determine the minimal percentage gross profit you need and consistently generate enough lab work to achieve it, using as a reference the 50-percent return you can achieve on every test sent to a commercial lab.

If you currently own lab equipment, use these techniques to make sure the equipment is in profit compliance and monitor the results on a regular basis. If you are considering the purchase of lab equipment, use these techniques to analyze your situation and make sure it is the right business decision for your practice.

Adoption center management

by John Lofflin

"Pet adoption creates a lifelong partnership between the veterinarian, the pet and its adoptive family."

Marty Becker, DVM

The photos in the dusty album capture the family's most important moments and precious memories: births, marriages, college graduations—and the adoption of the family pet. Look closely at the last photo and you'll see mom and dad on one side, junior on the other and the family's new puppy in between. Behind them, a sign reads, "Total number of homeless or abandoned pets adopted to date—256," just like the sign at McDonald's.

This sign is displayed at Dr. Marty Becker's All Pet Complex and Health Center in Salt Lake City, out of which he runs his pet adoption program. Their slogan is: Celebrating and Protecting the Human-Companion Animal Bond™, and this message is carried out through the PETS™ program. PETS™ stands for Prevention, Education, Training and Socialization.

This concept is also promoted at Dr. Ross Clark's Affection Connection in Tulsa. Both centers offer attractive space for adoptions, provide medical care for the animals they take in and emphasize screening and education of the adoptive families. This concept straddles the fence between philanthropy and practice building.

What is a pet-adoption center and how does it work?

With their permission and assistance, I have used both Dr. Clark's Affection Connection and Dr. Becker's All Pet Complex as model adoption centers for this article.

Structure. The Affection Connection is a nonprofit organization. Woodland PetCare Centers lease space to the center, loans equipment to the organization, perform spays and neuters at reduced rates and provide other medical services. The Affection Connection is associated with private humane organizations in Tulsa that work with a network of area veterinarians.

Dr. Becker's pet-adoption program is part of his All Pet Complex and is housed and managed within the PETS™ center. The program is associated with Salt Lake County Animal Services, a division of the police department. The county conducts owner-selection interviews and handles the corresponding paperwork.

Facilities. The All Pet adoption area covers about one-fourth of the 7,000-square-foot hospital. It requires one coordinator and two additional staff members. The center is open 12 hours a day, seven days a week. Dr. Becker's description: "State-of-the-art."

Both facilities can best be described as showcases. The cages are open; the areas are well-lighted; and the atmosphere in each facility is warm and inviting. The Affection Connection has translucent cages back-lit with blue light giving them a clean, sparkling white appearance.

The adoption concept

The purpose of adoption centers is to place homeless animals with responsible families, with the emphasis on "responsible." If you just "hand out" animals, it's a disservice to everyone involved. Without client education and pet behavioral training, 25 percent of adopted pets will be returned within two years; 75 percent within four years. At the Affection Connection, an adoption contract requires a prepaid spay or neuter and obligates the owner to provide the animal with "the basics."

Screening. A person's first pet is one of the most powerful, positive, significant events in life. Adoption centers should help craft that experience. A person cannot just walk in and say, "Boy, that's a cute puppy. I want him." Adoptive families must go through a pre-purchase consultation. Then, if they pass the interview, they can pick up the pet the next day. This one-day waiting period gives the center time to fully screen the family and also helps reduce impulse adopting. The family needs to be committed to a lifelong relationship with the new pet. According to Barbara Pope of the Affection Connection, "Anyone looking for a random pet to toss out into the backyard is not going to leave with one. If that's what they're looking for, we tell them there's nothing here."

At first, people think adoption centers are like a retail store where they will get the hard sell: "Please, take one." No. Pope always tells people up front, "That's not my role at all. If I don't think it's a good match, I'll tell you." And she has done just that:

"I had a man come in with a little child, who insisted on this tiny puppy that would have been smashed in three days. I told him, 'You're going to have a really tough decision to make when you bring me a broken puppy. Your child is so active, and this puppy is only six weeks old and so tiny.' He said, 'Hmm.' I then said, 'I suggest you take this four-month-old puppy over here; it's much sturdier; it can get away.' He said, 'Yep, sounds like a better choice.'"

It's best to just kind of nudge them along and let them make the decision. If they've got three kids and they want to adopt a puppy, it's up to you to remind them, "Remember, this is like taking in another child."

Education. Adoption centers should not place an animal in a home if it does not appear to be a good match. However, rather than send people out the door, it is possible to create better homes through education. "If there's any kind of window for education, we'll jump at it," says Pope. The Affection Connection and Woodland PetCare Centers work together to promote both education and animal health. They strive to educate people so they'll be able to maintain their animals properly.

When a family with kids says, "I don't know what it is, but all of our pets seem to meet some early demise," Pope responds with,

"Can we talk for just a second?" When she gets to talk to them alone, she asks exactly what they meant. "They'll tell me one got in the dryer and got fried. Now, accidents happen; but let's just not take it lightly."

She goes on to say, "I've heard so many horror stories, I could write a book. It's amazing how many people come in and say, 'I'm looking for a cat.' When asked, 'What happened to the cats you've had before?' they say, 'Well, one got hit by a car; one got poisoned; one got shot.' So you say, 'Are you going to keep this one inside?' And they say, 'Well, no.'" This is a time for education, for a family conference about this problem.

Adoption centers should strive to create and strengthen the human-animal bond. Dr. Becker's program places adoptive families into a complimentary behavioral training seminar, where new pet owners are taught about how to deal with biting, barking, digging, chewing, scratching and litterbox training.

Each session of the behavior seminar is begun by encouraging new owners to reminisce. "We take them back on a mental journey to the first pet they had in their lives," says Dr. Becker.

"Then we talk to them about this unique bond they're going to have with this new pet. We want their relationship with the pet to be as enjoyable as possible.

"We've adopted out homeless pets in a cooperative program for eight years," says Dr. Becker, "but this program has taken it to a new level in which we take that episode, the adoption and celebrate it. The adoption episode is a lifelong partnership among the veterinarian, the pet and its adoptive family. We want to prevent as many problems as possible. We tell people we want this pet to be happy and healthy and live life to its fullest potential."

Behavior education is where you save lives; that's where you create responsible pet ownership. Five years ago, if you asked veterinarians to name the number one killer of dogs, answers would have been varied. Today, however, there is a growing consensus: The number one killer of dogs in the U.S. is euthanasia resulting from behavior problems. There is a tremendous behavioral awareness now. We know the problem. We have just chosen through neglect or indifference not to do much about it.

"The public wants veterinarians involved in the whole ecosystem of the animal," Dr. Becker says. The human-animal bond is gaining in importance as societal, neighborhood and family relationships break down. If that bond is gaining in importance and the number one killer is euthanasia, it makes sense that we address behavioral problems and that we "celebrate and protect the human-companion animal bond™."

Most behavior problems are minor if we catch them early on. "Everybody has in mind this puppy they're going to get for the kids that will sleep in the house, on the bed," says Arlo Brown, operations manager at All Pet Complex. "Suddenly it starts growling, starts getting rambunctious; it's biting the kids; it's soiling all over the place. They can't deal with it; so they throw it in the backyard. It's barking there; it's digging; it has an increased stress level. That's not a positive relationship. A situation like that doesn't benefit the client, the pet or the hospital."

To avoid situations like this, All Pet Complex strives to foster the concept that pets are a part of the family. They strive to prevent as many problems as possible. It is always better to have adoptive families bring in pictures of their pets for the family album in the adoption center than bring in their pets because of behavior problems. Dr. Becker says, "We want to prevent as many problems as possible. That demonstrates that we're different from the typical 'treat-accidents-and-illnesses' practice. Rather, we want to be involved in a leadership position for the pet's entire ecosystem."

Dr. Becker's practice philosophy is reflected in every activity in the hospital. Education is the best way to create a lasting bond between owner, pet and veterinarian.

One client at a time

In addition to the synergism that adoption centers have with preventive medicine, adoption programs tap into another trend in modern veterinary practice.

According to Dr. Becker, this trend requires practice building one client at a time. The idea: to build a business and build better clients by reaching deeper into your client base–one client at a time–rather than constantly striving to make the client base wider.

The idea comes from a book called *The One to One Future ... Building Relationships, One Customer at a Time*, (New York: Doubleday, 1993), which talks about getting more of an individual client's market share versus a bigger share of the market. You're striving for 100 percent of your client's business. For a veterinarian, that means if you're going to be involved in adopting out an animal, then you want to be involved in helping with behavioral problems and with the entire ecosystem of the pet. You want to gain a larger share of a client's business, one client at a time.

Using All Pets Complex as an example, during its first year of operation the center has adopted out 215 animals, which translates into roughly 172 potential clients. According to Brown, more than 80 percent of adopted pets return to the practice for other services. The adoption center fits perfectly with veterinarians' desires to improve their client base. With an adoption center, you're able to create your own clients, bond with the clients you create and establish a lifelong relationship.

Staff morale

Another benefit of adoption centers is staff morale. Says Brown, "They feel the reward of working with abandoned and homeless pets from the community. Otherwise, the 215 pets we've placed would have been euthanized." Barbara Pope makes this observation: "One other benefit that may not register on a practice's bottom line right away is the good feeling these centers create among staff members." The personal satisfaction gained from a successful adoption is immeasurable.

Pope is proud to say, "People are always bringing their pets back just to visit. We take a personal interest in these animals, and the people know it. We get to know them; we get attached. The best thing in the world is when they bring them back for their boosters at Woodland, and they pop their heads inside our office and say, 'Just wanted to let you know we're over here.' Of course, you have to go over and squeal about how big the dog has gotten."

Dr. Becker says that his reward comes from seeing adoptive families bringing in pictures of their pets for the family album in the adoption center–pets that are now part of the family.

This article originally appeared as "Taking pet-adoption centers to new heights" in the September 1994 issue of *Veterinary Economics*. It is reprinted here by permission of the publisher.

Notes

Notes

Notes

Notes